THE PAIN-FREE BODY

SIMPLE **STRETCHES** AND **EXERCISES** FOR COMMON ACHES AND PAINS

DR. DAN GINADER, PT, DPT

First published in 2025 by Victory Belt Publishing, Inc.

ISBN-13: 978-1-628606-13-3

The information included in this book is for educational purposes only. It is not intended or implied to be a substitute for professional medical advice. The reader should always consult their healthcare provider to determine the appropriateness of the information for their own situation or if they have any questions regarding a medical condition or treatment plan. Reading the information in this book does not constitute a practitioner-patient relationship.

Cover design by Elita San Juan
Interior design by Charisse Reyes
Illustrations by Elita San Juan, Charisse Reyes, Alyanna Alcira, Crizalie Olimpo
Photography by Charles Henry

Printed in Canada
TC 0125

This book is dedicated to my mother, who took out a second mortgage on her home so I could afford to go to PT school.

This book is also dedicated to the love of my life, Sable. Without her support and encouragement, I likely would have never had the confidence to create content or write this book.

FOREWORD

There are people who change the way you think. And then there are people who change the way you move. Dr. Dan Ginader did both for me.

When you're chasing a world record, there's very little room for error. Every hour, every step, every decision matters. After finishing my first Ironman—the first of six in my world record attempt—my body broke down. I was in pain, limping, and unsure if I'd even make it to the start line of my second race in Australia, just thirty days later.

I had already seen numerous physical therapists. No one could figure it out. Time was running out, and hope was wearing thin. I wasn't just looking for relief—I needed a miracle. I needed someone who could look past the symptoms.

That's when I flew across the country to see Dan in person.

In a single session, he pinpointed the exact root of the issue—no guesswork, no generic fixes. Just precision, experience, and intuition. He didn't just treat the pain. He explained it. He showed me how to move differently, how to understand my body better, and how to trust the healing process.

Over the weeks that followed, we worked together virtually to not only manage the injury, but completely resolve it. Not only did I make it to the start line—I crossed the finish line seventeen minutes faster than my first race.

What could've been a season-ending injury became a minor detour. And that's the power of what Dan teaches in this book.

Dan's superpower is not just his clinical expertise—though he has that in spades. It's his ability to listen deeply, simplify the complex, and empower you to heal with your own two hands. He doesn't throw generic protocols at you. He customizes. He explains. He helps you believe in your own body again. He didn't just help me get back to racing—he reminded me that pain doesn't have to be where the story ends. Sometimes, it's where the strongest chapters begin.

The Pain-Free Body is more than a guide—it's a gift. A manual for people who are tired of band-aid solutions and are ready to feel better—not just once, but for the long haul. Whether you're training for an Ironman, chasing a big dream, or simply want to move through your day without discomfort, this book is your toolkit for sustainable relief and lasting strength.

Dan kept me on the path to chasing my goals. Now, he's giving you the tools to chase yours.

Because you don't just deserve to be pain free—you deserve to feel like yourself again.

— Ariana Luterman, 2-Time IRONMAN® Triathlon World Record Holder

CONTENTS

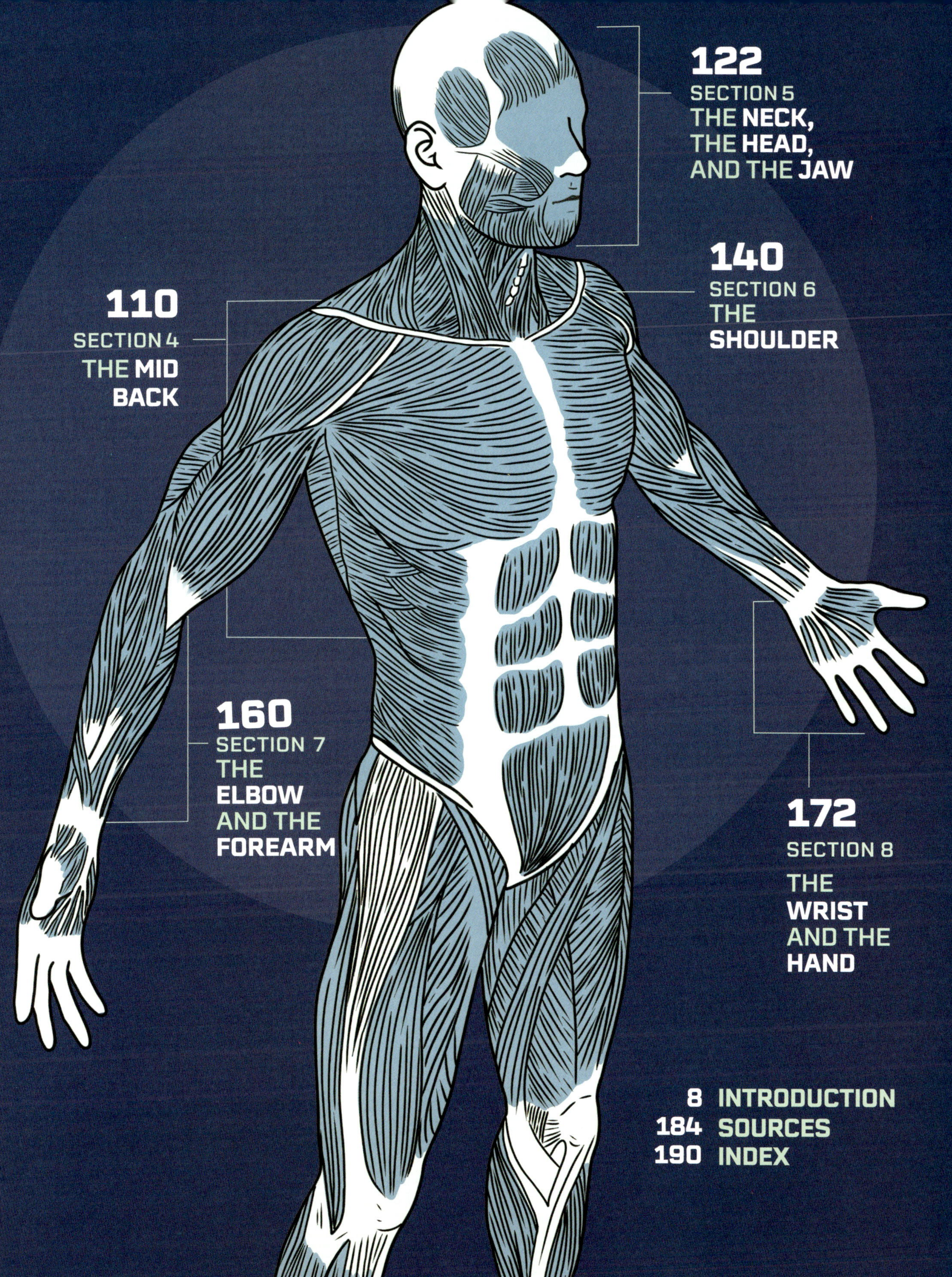

INTRODUCTION

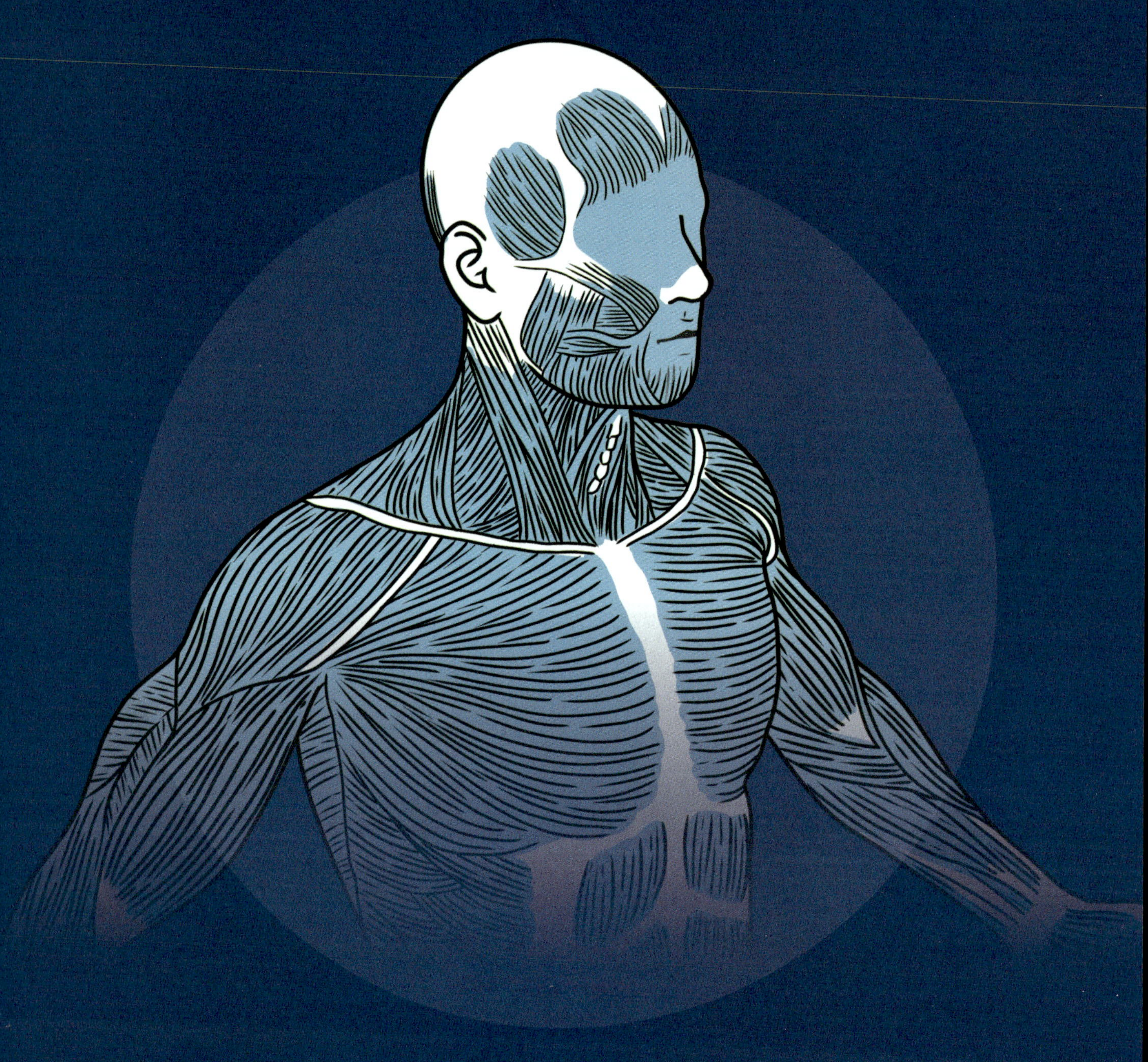

My name is Dan Ginader, also known as Dr. Dan, DPT. I am a Doctor of Physical Therapy who (at the writing of this book and hopefully for much longer) practices at Mims Method PT in the heart of New York City. The journey to writing this has been kind of a wild ride, but I believe that this book is the best way to continue the work that I have been doing and to help as many people as possible.

In early 2020, I was practicing as the physical therapist inside the State Government Center of Indiana. I had been recruited to work for a company called Tx: Team, which specialized in opening private PT clinics inside large corporate offices. I started in December of 2019, and within my first two weeks, I was booked SOLID. I was convinced that this was the future of physical therapy: Going to where the people are, being in network with their insurance, and offering one-on-one care at an affordable price. It couldn't have been going better.

Then, as some of you may remember, the world ended. In March of 2020, I went from being fully booked to all of a sudden having absolutely nobody on my schedule. Being a PT in an office building went from being the best job in the world to basically no job at all.

By the time May rolled around, I hadn't treated a patient in a couple of months, and I had also developed a crippling TikTok addiction. One week, I kid you not, I spent forty-two hours on the app just consuming videos. After having a "come to Jesus" talk with myself, I decided that I either needed to delete the app and see a therapist or find a way to make it a productive use of time.

And so, I posted my first TikTok under the handle @dr.dan_dpt. After a few weeks, one of my exercise videos set to a popular song at the time went viral, and the rest is history. By continuing to post simple stretches and exercises, in about four years I had over a million followers across all social platforms.

As my online content and presence have continued to grow, one thing has never stopped surprising me: Every single week, without fail, I get comments and messages telling me how a video that I made helped someone get out of pain. To me, as a PT, these videos are nothing but very simple pieces of information that are basic enough to apply to large groups of people. And yet, this very simple information is all people need to really make a difference in their lives.

As I've grown both as a PT and as an educator, I have continued to look for more ways to spread this simple information to help people relieve the pain that they have grown accustomed to living with. Through that, *The Pain-Free Body* was born. In this book, I take an in-depth look at the principles behind my videos, and I include a lot of diagnoses and exercises that I have never talked about before.

This book will not offer a magic cure for every ache and pain that you will have—that should go without saying. But by using nothing more than the information in this book, a lot of people will feel significantly less pain, and, at the very least, they will start their journeys to becoming pain free by learning about their bodies and taking steps in the right direction.

HOW TO USE THIS BOOK

Welcome to day one of physical therapy! When I see someone for the first time, I have three main goals for that initial visit:

1. Find out what is causing their pain
2. Figure out something that I can do to create at least some immediate relief from that pain
3. Identify two or three movements that the patient can start doing on their own to begin the journey of fully resolving their pain

My hope is that I have effectively shared my thought process when it comes to these diagnoses and made them simple to understand. This book covers the most common causes of aches and pains that I have seen throughout my career and shares the movements, techniques, and advice that I have given those patients. If you are struggling with an ache or pain, you will hopefully be able to align with one of the listed causes and then have immediate access to exercises that have successfully worked for people struggling with that type of pain.

My vision for this book is that you will keep it around the house the same way that you would keep ibuprofen on hand: You almost forget you have it until the second that you need it, and then you can quickly find it and use as needed.

For instance, if you are experiencing knee pain, go to the section of this book dedicated to the knee. Find the area of the knee that most closely aligns with your symptoms and read about the possible causes of your pain. You may be referred from there to other places in the book, or you may be prompted to try the suggested techniques and movements, get a new understanding of your pain, and start feeling like you're moving in the right direction.

Always make sure that the suggested movements and exercises *do not* increase your symptoms. Err on the side of caution; it is better to feel like something is too easy or gentle than to push too hard, which could lead to increased symptoms. And trust the process. Symptoms of ongoing pain do not clear up overnight. It takes a lot of consistency and the belief that what you are doing will make a difference.

If you go through the recommendations and exercises in this book and your pain isn't resolved, then please don't hesitate to see a physical therapist in person. Basic information is great, but nothing beats the personal touch of a high-quality professional. While the techniques I go over in this book will work for a lot of common aches and pains, there are some diagnoses that require a more personal touch. If you are working on a particular pain for one to two weeks and haven't felt a difference, please see a professional in person to avoid any long-lasting issues.

Finally, and perhaps most importantly, this is a reference book. It is a collection of movements and exercises that I have seen work for things in my practice, but it is not a prescription. Without evaluating your pain in person, I lack the ability to provide any specific advice. But by reading through this book, you can see what diagnosis you may align with and learn about some stretches and exercises that have worked in other cases.

SECTION 1

THE FOOT, THE ANKLE, AND THE LOWER LEG

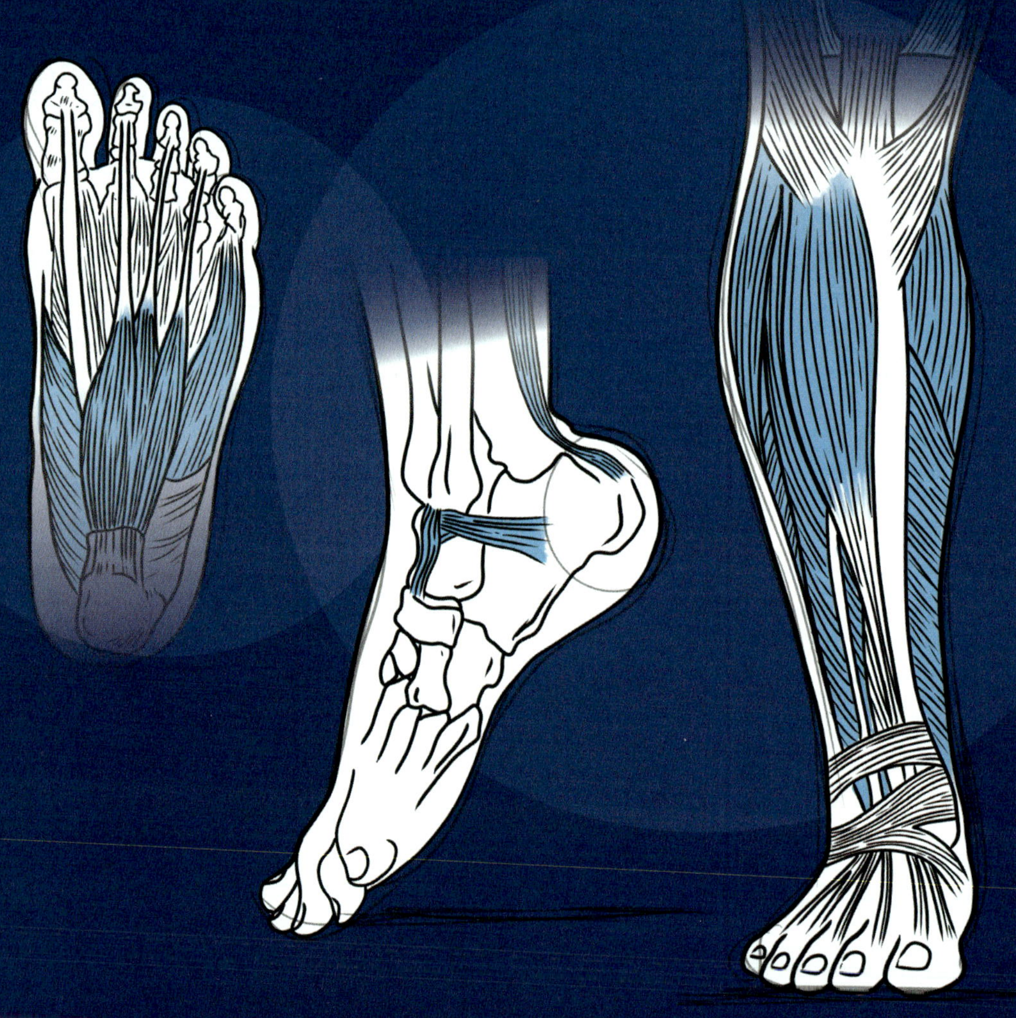

Foot and ankle injuries are among the toughest to deal with because so much of life requires us to be on our feet or to have our feet on the ground (e.g., sitting in a chair), so these injuries can take the longest to heal and cause a lot of frustration. The diagnoses and tips in this section are designed to address the problems at their sources and get you back on your feet (hopefully pain free).

THE BIG TOE

If you are reading this section, it means that you are experiencing discomfort in your big toe, and for that I offer plenty of empathy. The big toe is the part of the foot where the most action takes place. It is not only your primary source of balance and stability in the foot but also the last thing that leaves the ground every time you take a step.

In my time working with dancers, I have come across too many big toe issues to count, the most common of which are covered in this section. In a lot of cases, you can make massive differences in how the big toe feels without ever technically addressing the big toe itself. By focusing your efforts on increasing flexibility in the ankle, you can remove a lot of stress from the big toe, and keeping stress off it allows it to heal.

If you lack flexibility in your calf and in the muscles of the bottom of the foot, the big toe has to take on a lot of extra work. Since it is the last thing to leave the ground, it is basically your last line of defense every time you take a step. And if the big muscles in your calf (the gastrocnemius and soleus) aren't holding up their end, the poor big toe is left with a payload it was never meant to handle. When that is the case for long enough, stress and strain build to the point of pain and lead you directly to this chapter.

WHAT TO DO FOR A STUBBED TOE

This book is mostly about chronic conditions: pain that has been around for a while that you aren't quite sure about where it came from, what is causing it, and what to do about it. This is not a book for what to do after something like stubbing your toe.

That being said, after telling my girlfriend that I had finished writing the section on the big toe, she said, "Great! Now people will know what to do after they stub their toe." So now I am writing this tangent for all of the people who just stubbed their toe.

Give it twenty-four to forty-eight hours, and if it is still really painful, try to stay off it and keep it elevated. After a couple of days, if it is still bothersome, return to this book and skip ahead to the Ottawa Ankle Rules [page 21], which will help you figure out if you have a fracture along with what to do if you do.

HALLUX RIGIDUS/LIMITUS

Even if you don't speak Latin, you can probably use context clues to figure out exactly what this diagnosis translates to. *Hallux* is the anatomical term for your big toe, and *rigidus* and *limitus* just translate to "rigid" and "limited" (I know, it's a big leap). Put as simply as possible, it is a degenerative condition that leads to extremely limited ranges of motion in the big toe itself. It normally involves some sort of arthritis or bone spurs that reduce how much mobility you have in the big toe. Hallux limitus is where the toe is very stiff, but you still have some ability to move the big toe, whereas rigidus is where you have next to none. Either way, it can be incredibly painful when pushing off the foot while walking or rising up to your tiptoes. It will not only feel like you don't have the mobility that you should, but you will also feel a lot of discomfort once you get to that end range.

Limited Range of Motion in the Big Toe

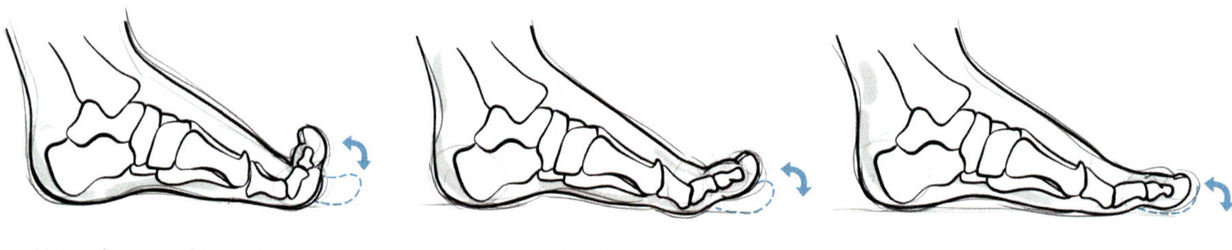

Normal range of motion | Hallux limitus | Hallux rigidus

Since hallux rigidus/limitus is a degenerative condition of the joint, there is nothing that can be done to change what is actually happening in the big toe, outside of a surgical procedure to shave down a bone spur if that is the main limiter. But just because there is nothing that can technically be done to change the anatomical structure, that doesn't mean there is nothing that you can do to decrease symptoms.

In the past year alone, I have treated two high-level Broadway performers with symptoms that align with hallux limitus, and they have been able to keep dancing on stage eight times a week, mostly by following the movements you can find in the "Self-Massage" and "Stretches" sections beginning on page 38.

It also helps to limit any action that causes a sharp increase in symptoms until your symptoms abate. This may include things like running or even something like rising up on your toes in bare feet. Since the main course of treatment is to reduce strain over the long term, symptoms may take a while to clear, so it's a good idea to try to limit stress and strain where possible.

It can also be helpful to wear forgiving shoes with a wide toe box, a rocker sole, and thick padding. Thick-soled rocker bottom shoes have been a favorite for people dealing with this condition.

FLEXOR HALLUCIS LONGUS TENDINITIS/TENDINOSIS

If you aligned with the painful symptoms of hallux rigidus/limitus but feel like you still have a lot of range of motion, you may be dealing with an issue in the tendon of your flexor hallucis longus (FHL). (If you're wondering whether you lack range of motion in the big toe, just compare the motion of the toe to its counterpart on the other foot. In general, this is a good principle to follow for all pains. If the painful side moves just as much as the non-painful side, then you likely aren't lacking range of motion.)

If you read the last section, you already know that *hallucis* is just Latin for the big toe. *Flexor* simply denotes that this is the muscle that flexes (bends) the big toe, and *longus* means that it is the longer of the two muscles that do that. (There is also a brevis muscle that is largely unproblematic.)

If this tendon really is your source of discomfort, you will feel pain toward the bottom of the big toe or even up on the inside of your lower leg when pushing off while taking a step or rising up on your toes. Whereas with hallux rigidus, a lot of the symptoms are on the top side of the toe.

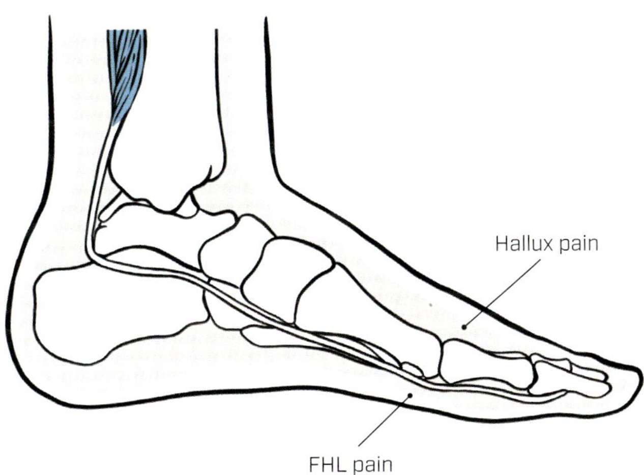

The main cause of irritation in this muscle and tendon can be a lack of flexibility in the calf, and the treatment is largely the same as it is for hallux rigidus/limitus. This diagnosis just has a better long-term outlook since there is no degeneration in the joint itself.

See the "Stretches" section on page 39 and progress to the "Exercises" on page 40 when you get to the point where you can rise up on your toes with minimal discomfort.

BUNIONS

Believe it or not, bunions aren't just for grandparents! A bunion is a bony bump on the outside of your big toe that causes your big toe to point toward your second toe and ultimately pushes the rest of your toes toward the outside of the foot. The "bump" of the bunion can be incredibly painful to the touch due to inflammation. Bunions can come for anyone, though they are more common in elderly women than any other demographic. One of the main contributors to bunions is the consistent pressure of a narrow toe box (more common in women's shoes, especially heels) over a long period of time.

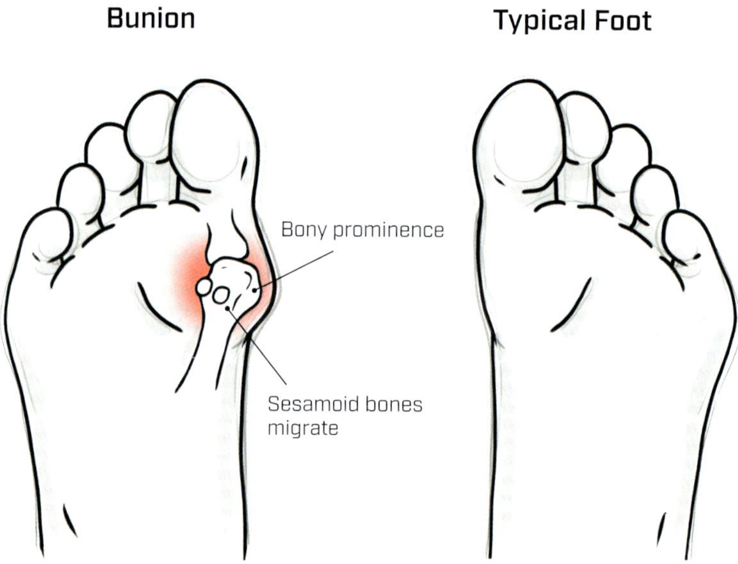

Unfortunately, once the bunion has formed, there is not much that can be done to reverse it outside of a surgical procedure. A bunionectomy can be incredibly uncomfortable and has varying results, which is why it is important to catch a forming bunion early and prevent it from getting worse. Therefore, it is important to build as much flexibility and strength as possible while also removing the stress of tight and narrow shoes.

While there are of course many other factors at play, chiefly genetics and age, the best first step in treating bunions is to trade in narrow shoes for something much wider at the toes that allows the feet to breathe a little bit. It also helps to follow the techniques listed in the "Stretches" section on page 39 to take stress away from the big toe. Once symptoms reduce in the big toe, you can begin the movements in the "Exercises" section on page 40.

With the right combination of shoes and exercises, even though a small bump or bunion will remain present on the outside of the big toe, painful symptoms can be reduced to the point where surgery is (hopefully) not needed.

SESAMOIDITIS

Unless you injure them, you would never know it, but in the pad that lies right underneath the base of your big toe, you have two very small, egg-shaped bones called sesamoids. These bones can become irritated and inflamed either slowly over time by repeated stress to the area or after you do something like landing from a height directly on that area.

Sesamoiditis

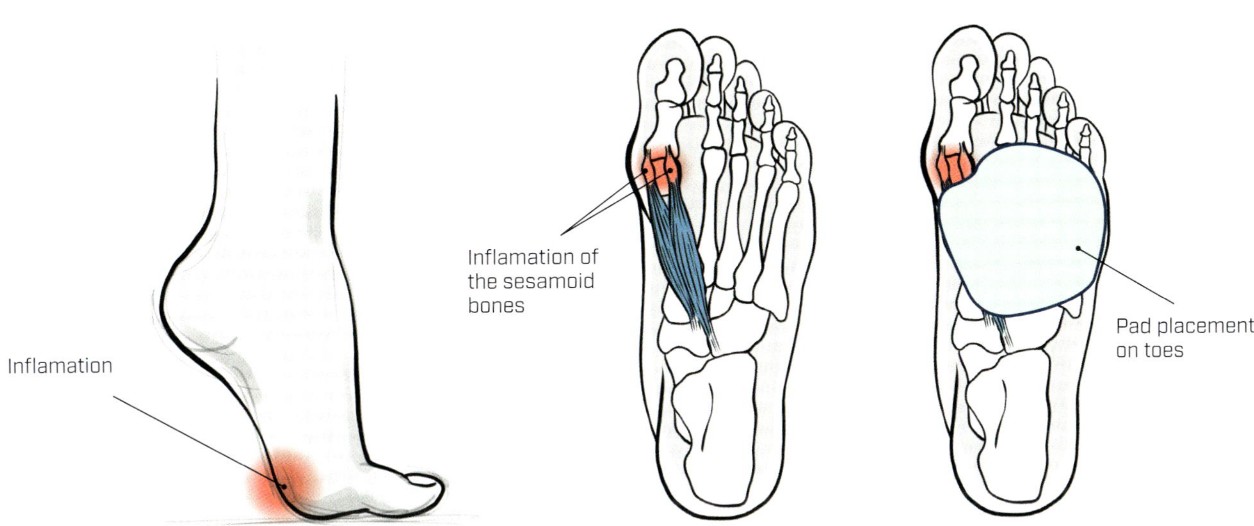

When you are suffering from sesamoiditis, putting weight on that area of the foot can be almost unbearable, and since that is an important area of your foot in terms of day-to-day function, it can take a while for things to calm down.

Much like the other big toe diagnoses, the best place to start is with the "Stretches" section on page 39 to begin to relieve the amount of pressure in the big toe. But for sesamoiditis, you can also purchase a product called sesamoid pads. These pads are mostly designed to stick directly to the bottoms of your feet to take weight off the sesamoid bones themselves. Using them during times when you have to walk or be on your feet prevents further inflammation from building while you continue to work on improving your flexibility.

THE REST OF THE TOES

I once had a patient who presented to me with foot pain and who had already seen multiple MDs and PTs to try to address it. Everything that she had tried revolved around the foot—basically everything suggested at the end of this section—and nothing worked. Since she had already tried everything, I decided to only work on her lower back and only give her movements for the lower back and the hips. After just four weeks, she had finally gotten the relief that she spent months looking for, and we didn't even look at her feet.

If you're experiencing regular discomfort in the rest of the toes or along the base of the rest of the toes, the fix may be as simple as getting shoes with a wider toe box. Especially if you frequently experience that discomfort after wearing a certain pair of shoes, your toes may literally just be getting squished. Along with wearing shoes with a wider toe box, you can use toe spacers for a few hours at the end of the day after getting out of your shoes to even out the compression that the toes have been experiencing. When buying toe spacers, just make sure you buy ones that are U-shaped or open ended. Toe spacers that encircle the toes won't fit everyone and can even exacerbate your toe discomfort.

However, if you are experiencing pain or especially numbness in the toes or along the foot that you don't feel has been addressed, please go to the chapter on the lower back where the dermatome map is discussed (page 97). Numbness, tingling, and even burning discomfort are most likely caused by nerve irritation higher up the chain of the leg, as far up as the lower back. It is still useful to follow the movements in "Stretches" (page 39) at the end of this section, but you should also be addressing the nerve pain with the movements outlined in the lower back section.

MORTON'S NEUROMA

While pain is often multi-factorial and hard to trace to one specific area, you may find yourself dealing with something very specific, like a Morton's neuroma. A Morton's neuroma can appear between either the second and third toes or third and fourth toes and can cause a numbing or burning pain that is hyper-localized to the area of the neuroma and worsens with tight shoes, particularly heels or shoes with narrow toe boxes, or when the area of the neuroma is compressed.

The neuroma itself is a thickening of the nerve tissue that has developed from consistent compression of the area. The small nodule will be inflamed and will also reduce the amount of space in the area, leading to pain and discomfort.

Therefore, the main fixes are to avoid shoes that increase compression, spend more time barefoot, and use toe spacers to relieve the compression. Often, as long as you're diligent about avoiding compression, the symptoms of the neuroma will clear up on their own. It also helps to follow the movements in the "Self-Massage" and "Stretches" sections on pages 38 and 39 to reduce overall stress in the foot.

But in cases where the neuroma is more stubborn and is not responding to the techniques listed here, you may need to see a surgeon for excision of the inflamed tissue.

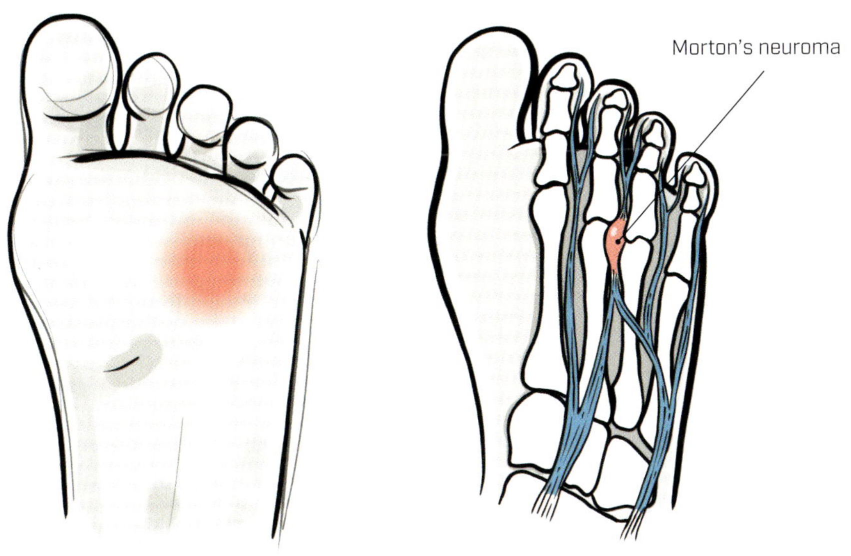

THE OUTSIDE OF THE FOOT/ANKLE

If what you are feeling along the outside of the foot is a burning, tingling, or numbness, especially if it extends to the outside of your lower leg, please read the section on the dermatome map on page 97. There is a high chance that your discomfort is coming from nerve irritation higher up the chain.

If what you're feeling is more of a tightness and stiffness that doesn't align with the diagnoses outlined below, please also read the section on plantar fasciitis on page 28. While plantar fasciitis presents most often in the plantar fascia, the heel, and the muscles in the arch of the foot, sometimes the muscles on the bottom of the outside of the foot can have a similar presentation, and by following the same tips and focusing on the outside of the foot, you can see similarly positive results.

FIFTH METATARSAL FRACTURE

The most common cause of localized pain on the outside of the foot is a fifth metatarsal fracture. Your fifth metatarsal is the bone that extends behind your pinky toe and runs along the outside of your foot. Due to its positioning and the size of the bone, it is one of the most fractured bones in the body. Sometimes it is fractured because of a traumatic event, like jumping down from a high platform or landing aggressively on the outside of the foot. But many times, it develops over time from overuse and forms as a stress fracture. This is most often the case in people who spend a lot of time on their feet or are avid runners.

Since this fracture is mostly developed over time, the symptoms can be slow to develop but will consistently worsen as you spend time on your feet. The main symptom is most commonly a deep achiness on the bottom side of the outside of the foot that doesn't respond to anything other than getting off your feet.

If you still aren't sure if you have a fracture, you can follow the Ottawa Ankle Rules on page 21 to point you in the right direction. If you think you may have a fracture in your fifth metatarsal, the only way to know is to see an MD and get an X-ray. In the event of a fracture, you will likely have to spend time in a walking boot or cast until the fracture has been given enough time to heal. If you don't have a fracture, then you can follow the advice listed in the "Ankle Sprains" section (page 22) since the recovery process will be very similar.

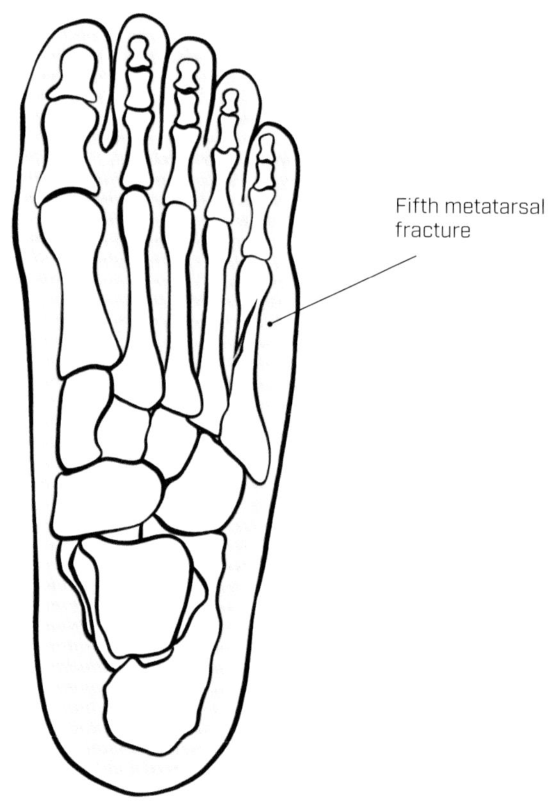

OTTAWA ANKLE RULES

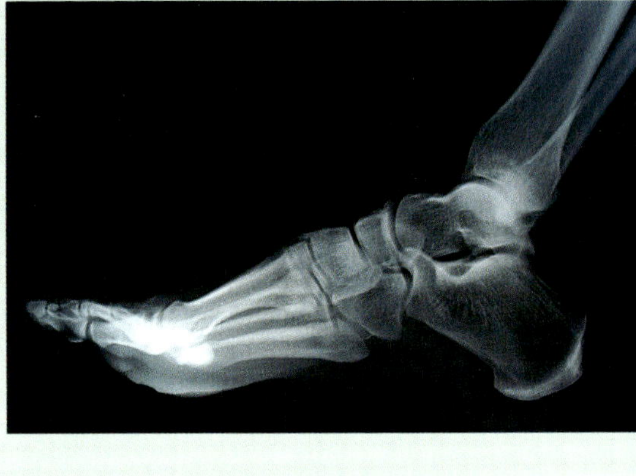

The Ottawa Ankle Rules were developed as an easy set of markers to use to determine whether somebody needs an X-ray when they present at a clinic. If you ever have a fall or some other incident that results in trauma to your foot or ankle, you can use these same five markers to help you decide whether you need to go and get imaging or it's something that you can manage at home.

The markers are:

1. Tenderness along the lower part of the back of the fibula or the tip of the lateral malleolus (outer ankle bone)
2. Tenderness along the lower part of the back of the tibia or the tip of the medial malleolus (inner ankle bone)

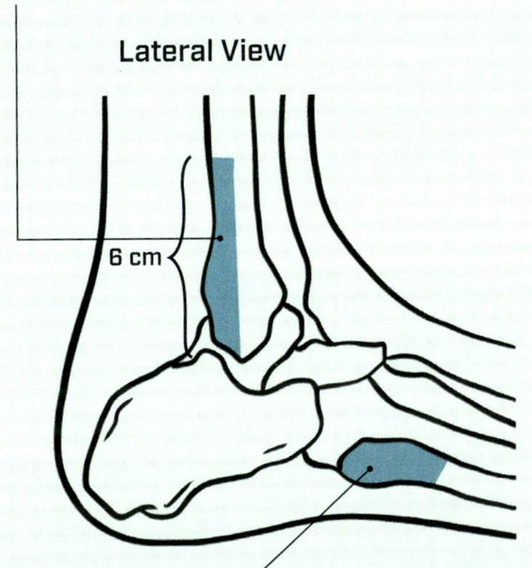

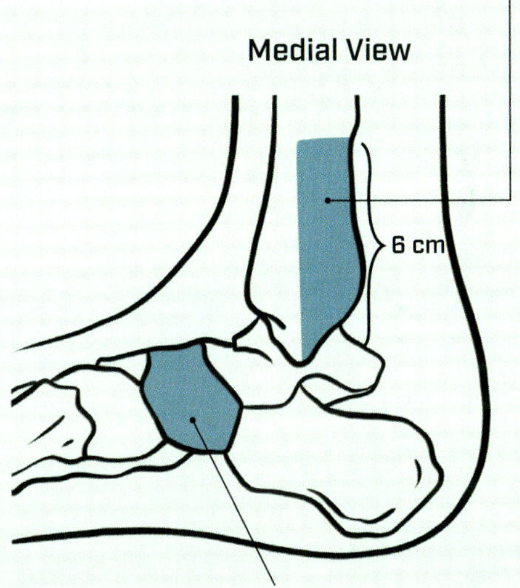

3. Tenderness along the base of the fifth metatarsal (outer part of the foot)
4. Tenderness in the navicular bone (pictured)
5. An inability to bear weight immediately after the injury or to bear weight for more than four steps twenty-four to forty-eight hours following the initial injury

If your injury presents with two or more of the five rules, then you qualify for a foot or ankle X-ray.

It is important to note that another hallmark sign of a fracture is extreme swelling and bruising along the foot and ankle. In late 2022, while playing football, I twisted my ankle trying to make a catch and felt immediate pain. Being a PT, I tried to just treat the injury myself. I didn't really have anything that I would consider overly tender, and I had the ability to bear weight and walk on it (albeit very uncomfortably), so I didn't fall under the Ottawa Ankle Rules. I did, however, have extreme swelling and bruising in my ankle and foot. After a week, it was still very painful, so I got an X-ray and found out that I had a complete but stable fracture along the bottom of my fibula. So, even if you don't meet the marks of these rules, don't ignore swelling, bruising, and continued discomfort, and just go in for imaging.

ANKLE SPRAINS

Ankle sprains come in all shapes and sizes, but they are all treated in much the same way. The overwhelming majority of ankle sprains occur on the outside of the ankle and are known as lateral ankle sprains. These generally occur after doing something like "rolling" your ankle outward after taking a misstep. The most commonly injured ligament is the anterior talofibular ligament (ATFL), but if you really did a number on yourself, you also may have injured the calcaneofibular ligament (CFL) and the posterior talofibular ligament (PTFL). The more ligaments that are affected, the longer the recovery process is likely to be.

The two less common forms of ankle sprains are known as medial ankle sprains and high ankle sprains. A medial ankle sprain may occur if your foot rolls inward while taking a step. This is a far less common injury because you have a lot less range of motion in that direction, making your ankle much more stable and harder to injure in that way. Also, the ligament on the inside of the ankle, the deltoid ligament, is far stronger than the three ligaments on the outside of the ankle.

High ankle sprains occur in the ligaments that connect the fibula to the tibia in the lower leg. They most often occur when the foot is planted on the ground and the lower leg rotates without the foot moving. The recovery process for high ankle sprains often takes the longest because of the area of the injury and because just bearing weight can strain it. With the other two forms of ankle sprains, you really need to strain the ankle inward or outward to irritate it, but just bearing weight is fine.

Luckily, no matter what form of ankle sprain you have, you can follow the same road map to recovery. The timeline will just vary based on the severity of your injury.

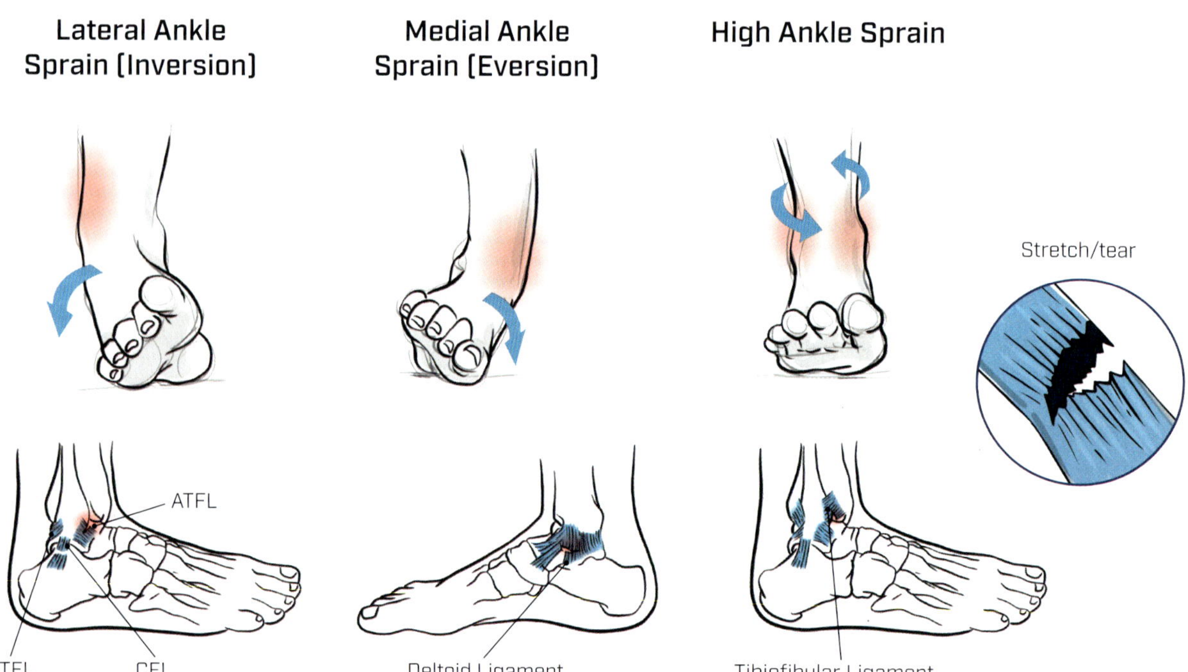

STEP 1: REST AND PROTECT

The rest phase may sound easy, but it does take a lot of patience since almost everything we do takes place on our feet, and it can be hard to allow yourself the time to properly rest the injured ankle.

As much as possible, you should be resting with the leg elevated above your heart. This will allow for better blood flow in the ankle and will limit excess swelling. If you are experiencing a lot of swelling, it is also a good idea to use a compression sock to help your body naturally circulate more swelling out of the ankle. It is no longer advised to use ice on something like an ankle sprain. Research has shown that ice constricts the blood vessels in an injured area and can actually slow healing.

If you do need to do something on your feet, make sure you are "protecting" the injury. Basically, don't do anything to irritate symptoms or swelling. Anything you can do without increasing symptoms or swelling, you are free to do. But pushing the ankle too far too soon can keep the injury irritated and prolong the healing time.

Once you have gotten to the point of your rest/protect phase where the ankle is feeling better and you can start to move it without increasing pain, then you can move on to Step 2.

STEP 2: RESTORE FLEXIBILITY AND MOBILITY

The movements and exercises for this phase are detailed at the end of this section, starting on page 39. But it is important to keep the movements fairly gentle. The goal is to push the ankle into as much range of motion as you can, but to be sure the movement is still comfortable and doesn't increase symptoms. Instead, just take what the ankle is giving you, and you will notice that every day will start to get a little easier and you will naturally be able to go further and further in your recovery.

If you are doing a good job keeping the movements gentle and not increasing symptoms, feel free to do these movements on a daily basis. Once you have the ability to do most of these exercises pain free, you can progress to the next step.

STEP 3: IMPROVE STRENGTH AND BALANCE

The movements and exercises for this phase are detailed at the end of this section (page 39). Keep doing the movements from Step 2 on a daily basis, but now start adding in strengthening and balance exercises. As you're moving on to building strength and balance, it is even more important to keep things at a level that doesn't increase symptoms. There should be minimal to no pain when moving through the exercises themselves, and ideally no pain in the immediate hours following. (It is, however, normal to feel some muscular soreness twenty-four to forty-eight hours after doing the exercises, especially the first few times.) You just want to make sure that the soreness isn't so significant that it limits your ability to move the ankle the next day.

Since these movements are more taxing than the previous step, it's best to start by doing them every other day. If you're noticing a lot of soreness, then stick to just two or three times a week. If you've gotten to the point where you feel little to no soreness, do them on a daily basis and move on to the fourth and final step.

STEP 4: RETURN TO ACTION

This step will look a little different for everyone since everyone's "action" is unique. If you play recreational basketball, this is when you can slowly start to jump and cut again. If you're a dancer, this is when you can slowly start to go through your classwork or choreography until you feel fully comfortable getting it back to 100 percent. If your highest level of action on a daily basis is walking around the block, this is when you can start to do that.

Whatever it is that you are returning to, just follow the same rules as the previous two steps. Start gently and don't allow your symptoms to increase. If there is soreness, allow yourself time to recover before getting back to it. Ultimately, build back at a sustainable rate and take what your body gives you.

If you follow these four steps as outlined, you should return to full force in the quickest and most efficient way possible.

FIBULARIS LONGUS/BREVIS TENDINOPATHY

If you are having pain on the outer ankle bone or along the outside of your foot that doesn't align with an ankle sprain or a fracture, then you may be experiencing an issue with the tendons of your fibularis longus and brevis muscles (formally known as your peroneal longus and brevis muscles). This muscle group originates in the outside of the lower leg and runs behind the outside of your ankle before attaching to the outside of the foot.

In isolation, it brings your foot into eversion (pointing the sole of your foot to the outside), but when you're weight bearing, it is a primary stabilizing muscle group for the foot and ankle. Especially if you have struggled with ankle sprains in the past, or if you feel like your ankle easily rolls inward, this muscle group can be under a lot of stress.

When this muscle group is irritated, you will feel stiffness and tightness anywhere along the path of the muscle or tendon, and you may find it hard to balance on the side of discomfort.

The best way to address this discomfort is to do the same exercises for strength and balance that you would do for an ankle sprain, focusing especially on the ankle eversion exercise. (See the stretches and exercises on pages 39 and 40.)

Once you build up the strength and endurance of the muscles, you should really start to notice a decrease in symptoms.

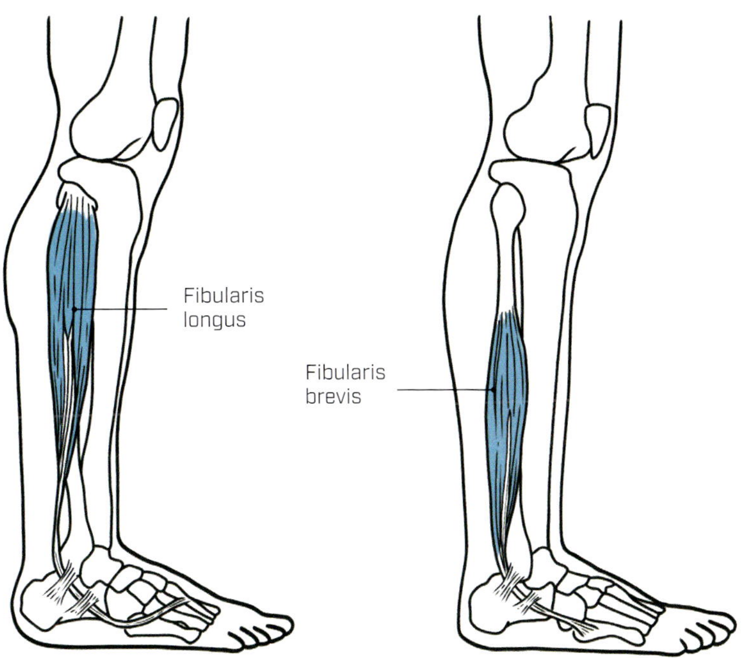

OTHER DISCOMFORT ON THE OUTSIDE OF THE FOOT

If the pain on the outside of your foot doesn't seem to align with anything mentioned in this section, be sure to also check the section about heel pain starting on page 26. Pain coming from the calf muscles most often presents in the Achilles area or bottom of the heel, but it can sometimes cause discomfort and stiffness along the side of the heel and the foot. Go straight to the section on Achilles tendon pain on page 29 and follow the suggested steps.

If addressing the Achilles tendon still doesn't seem to improve your symptoms, it is officially time to address your footwear. The most likely cause of nondescript discomfort in the foot is footwear that is either too narrow or not supportive. Try an over-the-counter orthotic to provide a little bit more support and wear shoes that are a little wider.

See the "Stretches" and "Exercises" sections starting on page 39 to help address symptoms as well. And if you find that you have tried everything in this section and nothing has done the trick, it is time to see a professional in person.

THE HEEL AND THE ARCH

The heel and the arch of the foot tend to go hand in hand. If you have read some of the other sections on the foot and ankle, you will have noticed a trend that increasing flexibility, especially into dorsiflexion (the ability to flex your foot toward your face), goes a long way toward relieving stress in the foot. Nowhere is that more the case than with pain in the heel or arch.

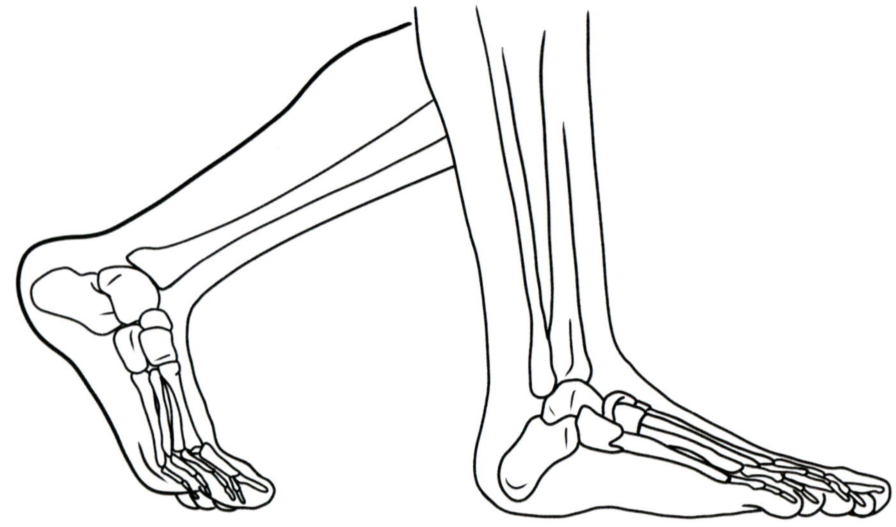

FLAT FEET

We are all born with flat feet, but in some people, the arch never develops, while others have an arch but develop flat feet over time. This is common in people struggling with obesity (body weight becomes too much for the arch to support, and it collapses) or diabetes (neurologic changes can lead to a condition known as Charcot foot). There is also something known as a "flexible" flat foot, which is when the foot shows a normal arch when off the ground, but the arch collapses when bearing weight. That can be caused either by the ligaments of the foot being too lax to support the arch or weakness in the muscles that support the arch itself.

The arch of the foot is a major shock absorber and allows for normal weight distribution further up the chain. The longer you go with minimal to no arch, the more wear and tear you will create in the foot and lower leg. If your flat feet are causing you discomfort, one of the first things you can try is placing an over-the-counter orthotic in your shoes. It doesn't need to be anything overly specific; generally, anything with a little extra support for the arch will help to alleviate symptoms. There are a few brands out there that offer great, affordable options. If you struggle to find an orthotic that's right for you, or you feel like you need something specific, you can always have a podiatrist make a custom one for you. (Spoiler alert: These are *much* more expensive.)

It is also important to build up the strength and flexibility in the foot by using the movements found at the end of this section on page 40. For this condition, while all of the movements are useful, it is best to focus on the exercises that work the tibialis posterior and the muscles of the arch of the foot.

For more information on the tibialis posterior, see "Posterior Shin Splints" in the lower leg section on page 33.

Typical Arch

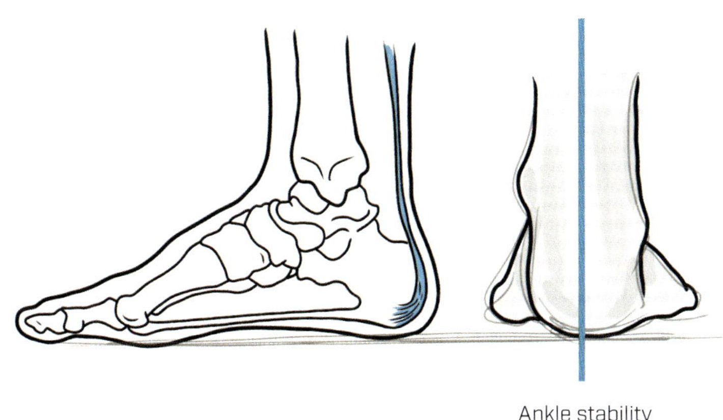

Ankle stability

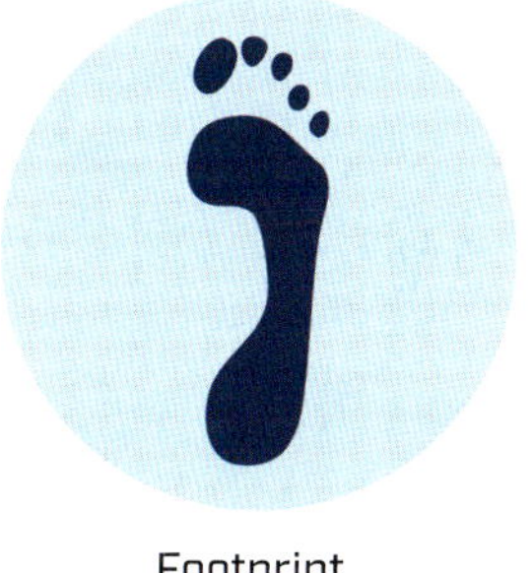

Footprint

Flat Arch

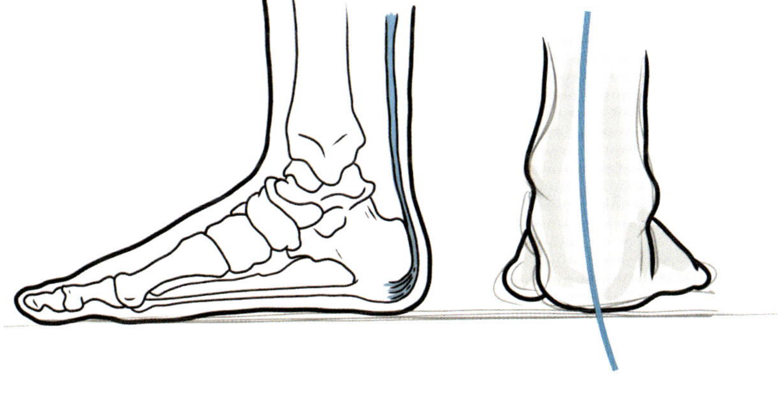

Ankle stability

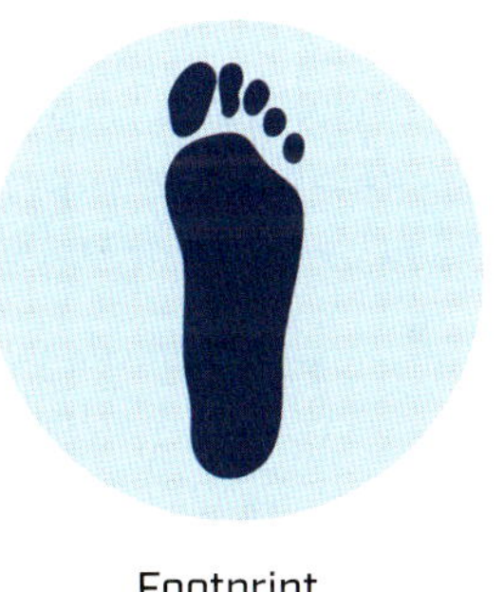

Footprint

PLANTAR FASCIITIS/FASCIOSIS

If I had access to the analytics of this book and could see which parts are the most read, I'm sure this would fall somewhere in the top five. So, if you're reading this, just know you are not alone.

Plantar fasciitis is an incredibly annoying condition. At its worst, it can make walking unbearable, and at best, it can make the first few steps of your day the worst part of your day. It occurs when there has been overuse in the arch of the foot over an extended period of time, affecting the plantar fascia (a band of tissue running from your heel to the base of your toes to support the arch) itself.

In its early stages, the pain will mostly be felt first thing in the morning, most likely on the bottom part of the inside of the heel where the plantar fascia starts. As it progresses, the pain will spread throughout the bottom of the foot, and symptoms will continue throughout the rest of the day. Eventually, it will begin to limit how much time you can tolerate walking or even standing. As with any foot or ankle diagnosis, it is best to start to address it as early as possible. Since symptoms worsen the longer you are on your feet, it can be challenging to deal with, especially if you're active.

Luckily, no matter what stage of this diagnosis you are in, it responds very well to physical therapy. By integrating the flexibility and strengthening movements at the end of this section, you can take strain away from the bottom of the foot, which will allow irritation to go down and symptoms to reduce.

All of the movements are important, but with plantar fasciitis, it's best to focus on the ball rolling (see page 38) and the calf stretching (see page 39) multiple times per day until symptoms start to reduce. As symptoms decrease, you can go down to just once a day, and eventually to just when you feel some tightness in the foot and calf. The strengthening exercises, however, are important to keep up two to three times a week until you have felt *zero* symptoms for at least two straight weeks. Since issues in the foot often recur, it's important to stay consistent to avoid the risk of a flareup.

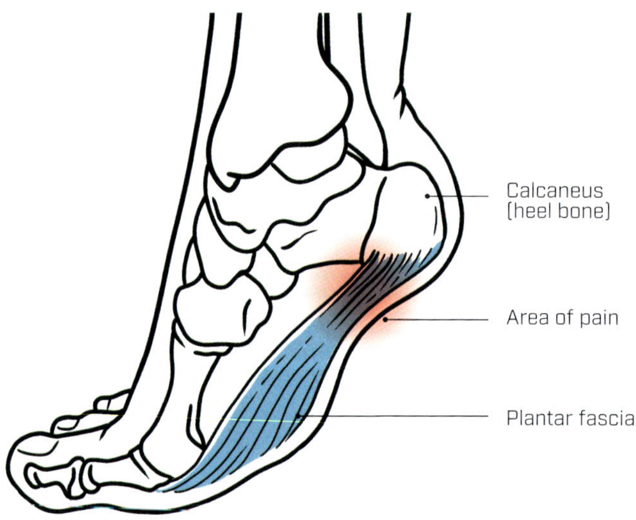

ACHILLES TENDINITIS/ TENDINOSIS

If you are having pain anywhere on the back side of your heel, it almost certainly is due to the Achilles tendon, since that is the only thing that attaches at that point. It is most common to feel the pain in the middle of the back of the heel, but you can also feel it on either side of the heel. No matter where in the back of the heel you are feeling the pain, the gastrocnemius (your bigger, more prominent calf muscle) and your soleus (the smaller, underlying calf muscle) are to blame, since those are the two main muscular attachments.

It is common for pain in this area to be worse first thing in the morning or after periods of inactivity. Stretching or walking can help loosen up the muscles and reduce symptoms, but if you try to do anything explosive, like run or jump, you may feel an increase in pain in the heel. If you let the pain progress, you may eventually get to the point where you are feeling pain in the back of your heel all the time, and not much can get it to calm down.

No matter what stage of the diagnosis you are in, it's important to start to improve the flexibility of the calf musculature. While it's a good idea to follow all of the suggestions starting on page 38, it would be good to focus mainly on the gastrocnemius stretch (see page 39) and the soleus stretch (see page 40). The goal is to find a gentle spot to hold the stretch where you can feel it in the muscle without an increase in pain in the back of the heel. If you are having trouble finding a stretch without pain, you can start by rolling out the calf with a handheld roller (see page 38). Once you get to the point where you can feel the muscle while doing the stretch, hold each stretch for twenty to twenty-five seconds and repeat three times. In the early parts of recovery, it's a good idea to do these stretches two or three times a day.

As flexibility begins to return and symptoms start to reduce, it is important to strengthen not just the muscles of the calf but the rest of the muscles in the foot and ankle as well. For the most part, the tightness comes from some form of weakness in the calf or overcompensation for other muscles in the lower leg. By addressing all of the areas, you can be sure that you are addressing the cause of your specific discomfort.

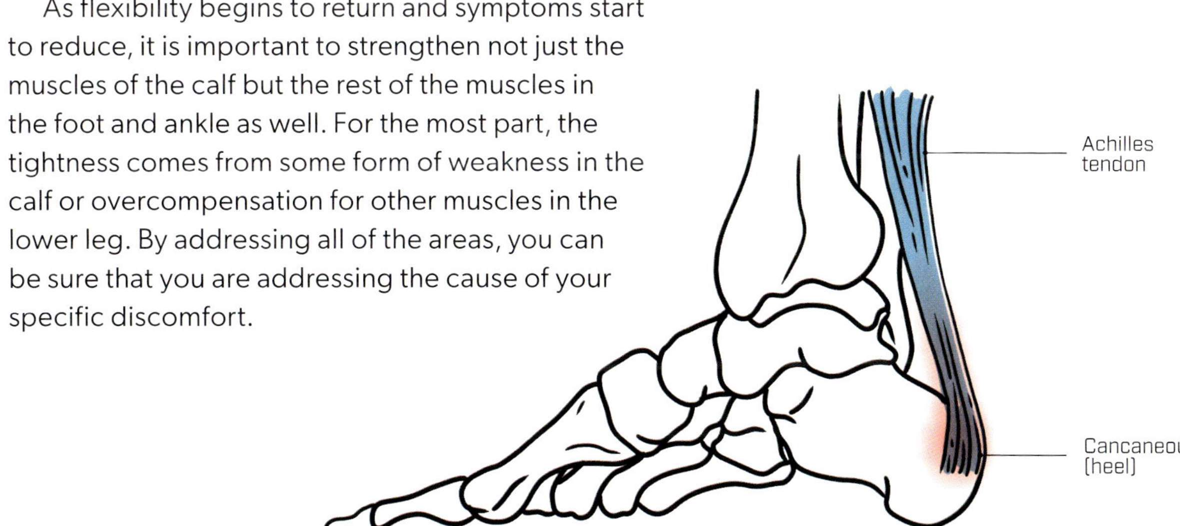

THE LOWER LEG

Most pain that comes from dysfunction in the muscles is felt where the tendons of those muscles attach to bone rather than over the muscle belly itself. Since all of the muscles in the lower leg have tendons that run down into the foot and ankle, it is worth looking into the previous section if you haven't already. The lower leg, foot, and ankle work together as one big unit, making it nearly impossible to improve one without also working on the other two.

While there are fewer conditions that create symptoms in the lower leg itself compared to the foot and ankle, when they are present, they can be debilitating. If you are a runner who has dealt with shin splints, or even just a fairly active person who has dealt with calf pain, you know exactly what I'm talking about.

When feeling discomfort in the lower leg, it can feel like you're walking through quicksand. You will go to move your ankle or try to push off the ground and feel like the ankle and foot are stuck and not listening to your simple instruction of just trying to move forward. Therefore, these lower leg injuries cannot be taken lightly.

SHIN SPLINTS

Shin splints come with two major presentations. One, referred to as "anterior shin splints," deals mostly with the tibialis anterior, and the pain is felt in the front of the shin. The other, referred to as "posterior shin splints," deals mostly with the tibialis posterior, and the symptoms are primarily on the inside of the lower leg and behind the shin.

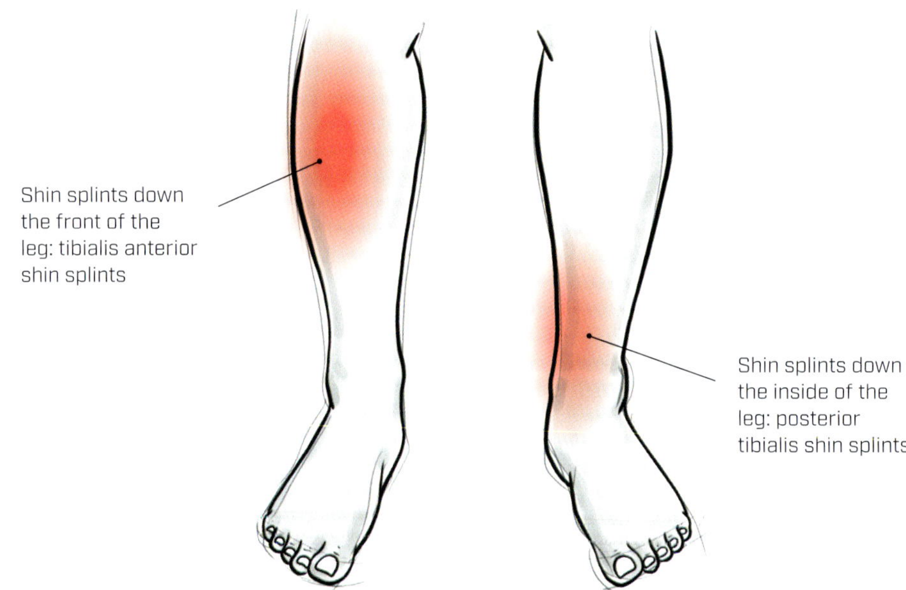

TA Causing Dorsiflexion

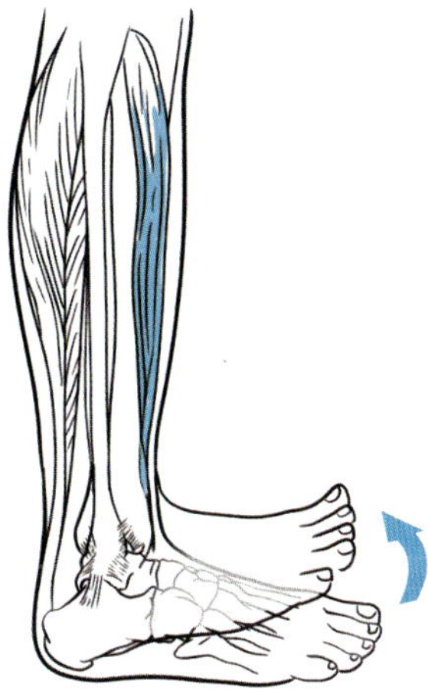

TA Pulling at the Tibia

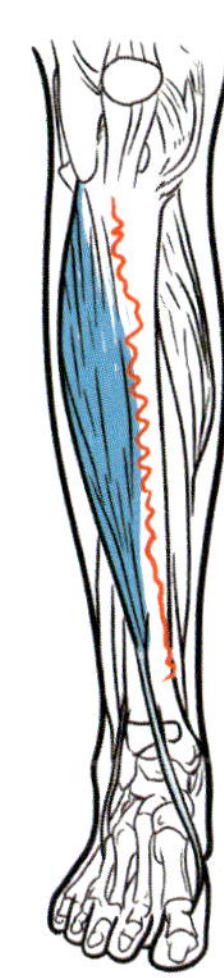

ANTERIOR SHIN SPLINTS

The most common cause of this diagnosis is overuse in a muscle called the tibialis anterior (TA). The primary action of this muscle is to create ankle dorsiflexion, or point your foot toward your face. Since it is necessary to get into ankle dorsiflexion while walking or running so your toes don't scrape across the ground, anterior shin splints have been known to pop up if you quickly increase the amount that you are doing either one of those two activities. If the tibialis anterior gets tight and irritated enough, it can start to pull at your tibia (shin bone) where it attaches along the length of the bone itself. When the symptoms build up to that point, just walking from your couch to your bathroom can become quite a chore.

While many factors can contribute to anterior shin splints, in my experience there are three main issues in people who are experiencing them:

1. A lack of ankle dorsiflexion
2. Weakness in the tibialis anterior
3. A tendency to land heavily on the heel when walking or running

Probably the most common theme among issues with the foot, ankle, and lower leg is that they can all be tied back into a lack of dorsiflexion, primarily due to a lack of flexibility in the muscles of the calf. In the case of anterior shin splints, the less dorsiflexion you have, the harder the tibialis anterior has to work in order to create that dorsiflexion. And until you improve the flexibility into dorsiflexion, the tibialis anterior will continue to be overworked and irritated just trying to do its job. To improve your dorsiflexion, focus mostly on the gastrocnemius and soleus stretches that are found at the end of this section. If you would like more information on the muscles that limit dorsiflexion, refer to the Achilles tendon section on page 29.

If there is overuse in a muscle group, that muscle is likely too weak to sustain the work that you are putting it through. And in the case of anterior shin splints, the weakness is primarily in the tibialis anterior. As you work on improving the flexibility into ankle dorsiflexion, you will also have to focus on building strength and control. The best exercise to accomplish this is the toe raises movement on page 42. Since this activates the muscle that is causing the symptoms, it is best to start with your feet fairly close to the wall and make sure you can complete at least three sets of ten with no increase in symptoms before making the exercise more challenging by moving your feet further from the wall.

As you improve your flexibility and strength in these two ways, your symptoms should start to improve over the course of a couple of weeks. But if you continue to land heavily on your heel, you may always be at risk of irritating this muscle group.

When you land on your heel, your tibialis anterior has to work incredibly hard to slowly lower your foot to the ground so you don't make a loud slapping noise every time you step. If you've ever turned heads with how loudly you run or walk on a treadmill, it is a sign that you are landing too heavily on the heel. Luckily, there is a mostly easy fix. If you are landing aggressively on your heel, it is probably because you are striding too far ahead of your center of gravity, making it difficult to land toward the middle of your foot. Simply by taking smaller but quicker steps, you can reduce strain on your tibialis anterior while moving just as fast.

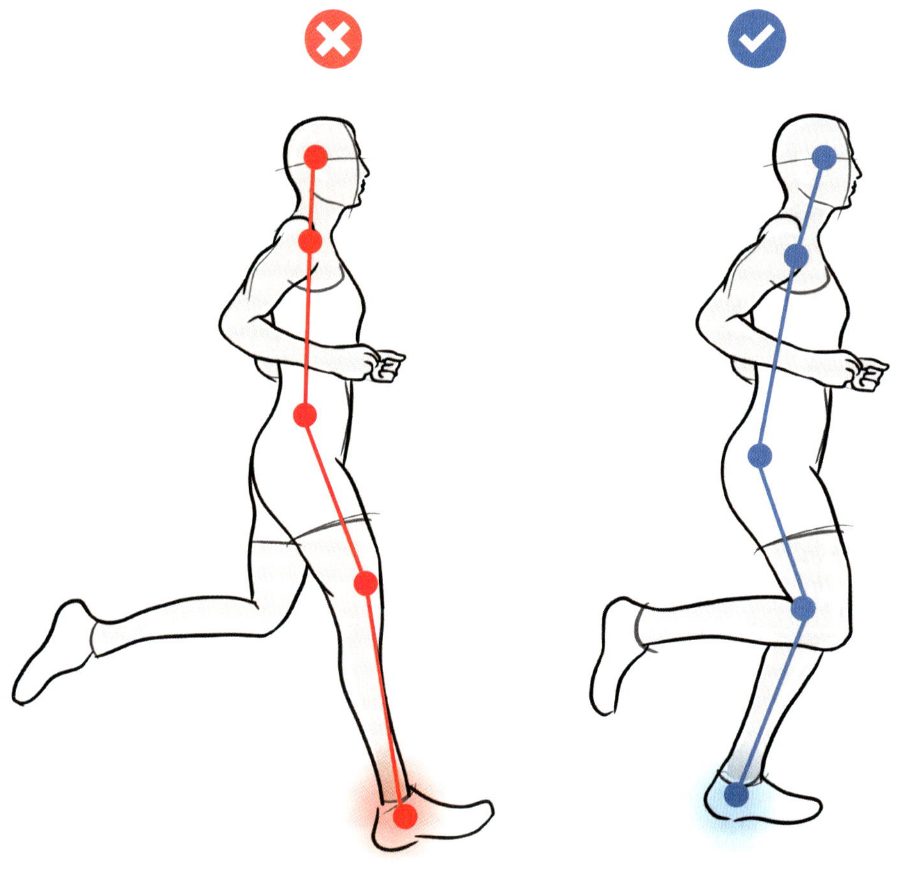

Heel Striking

Mid-Foot Strike

POSTERIOR SHIN SPLINTS

Posterior shin splints mostly create symptoms on the inside of and behind the shin bone, because that is exactly where the tibialis posterior lives. While this presentation is less common than anterior shin splints, it can be just as uncomfortable.

Since the tibialis posterior runs along the inside of the shin bone and down under the foot, it is most commonly overworked when the foot routinely falls into overpronation, or when the arch of the foot falls toward the floor. This is commonly the case when people with higher arches wear footwear with minimal arch support, which forces the muscle to work extremely hard to avoid that overpronation. For more information on this topic, refer to the section "Flat Feet" (see page 26).

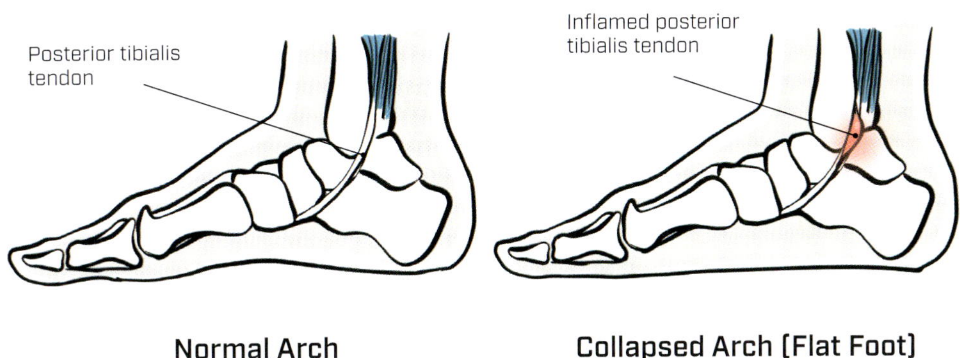

Normal Arch **Collapsed Arch (Flat Foot)**

Finding an insert to provide arch support can go a long way toward immediately reducing symptoms of posterior shin splints. But you also need to focus on building strength in the tibialis posterior to avoid overworking it while you walk or run. To do this, it is best to focus on the exercises at the end of this section that focus on the muscle, namely banded ankle inversion (see page 43) and the short foot exercise on page 44. Along with this, it is a good idea to focus on the exercises and stretches recommended for anterior shin splints.

THE OUTSIDE OF THE LOWER LEG

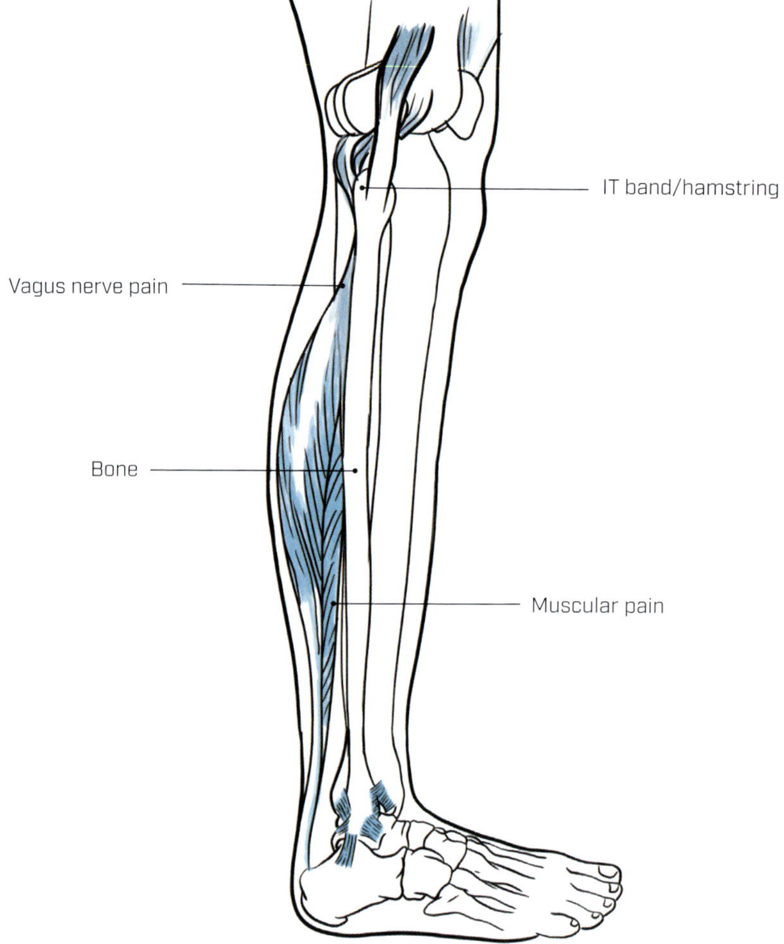

Pain along the outside of the lower leg can come from four main things:

1. The fibula, or the bone along the outside of the lower leg
2. Nerve pain coming from somewhere else higher up in the chain, such as your lower back
3. Muscular pain in the fibularis longus and brevis (see page 35)
4. Pain caused by the illiotibial (IT) band or hamstring attachment site (see page 63)

If you are feeling a burning and tingling sensation along the outside of the leg that doesn't seem to respond to anything you do to the area, refer to the dermatome map on page 97.

If you feel that the pain you are experiencing isn't described in this section and is mostly centered at the very top of the outside of the lower leg, then you might be dealing with number four, which is covered in the knee section (see page 63).

The two points covered in this section will be points number one and number three, since those are the two sources of pain local to the area.

FIBULA PAIN

The fibula is the long and skinny outer bone of the lower leg. Because it is fairly thin and positioned in a spot with minimal covering by any fat or muscle, it is a common place for fractures to occur. If you had a traumatic event recently in which you felt a painful pop, and especially if there was a lot of swelling and bruising, refer to the Ottawa Ankle Rules on page 21 to help you determine if you have sustained a fracture.

The fibula is also susceptible to stress fractures. These are most common in people who run a lot or spend a lot of time on their feet. If you have a dull and aching sensation that gets worse the longer you are bearing weight on the fibula, it is a good idea to get an X-ray to rule out a stress fracture, especially if it doesn't respond to the exercises suggested for the fibularis muscle group starting on page 42.

PERSONAL ANECDOTE

I fractured my fibula while playing flag football when I was twenty-nine years old. It swelled up and bruised like crazy, but I stubbornly tried to treat it myself for a week. It wasn't getting any better. I finally relented and got an X-ray, and sure enough, I had a complete fracture through the shaft of my fibula. Don't be like me! Get the X-ray sooner rather than later! This is the second time I've referred to this injury, so you know I'm serious.

FIBULARIS LONGUS/ BREVIS PAIN

These two muscles that run right along the fibula and down along the outside of the ankle were formerly known as the peroneal longus/brevis. When the muscle group is overworked and irritated, it can cause pain along the fibula, along with pain and weakness in the outside of the ankle.

The main difference in pain between this muscle and an issue with the bone is that the muscular pain responds very well to massage and exercise. If you massage the muscle group and do the exercises starting on on page 40 and feel a noticeable difference, then this is likely the source of your discomfort.

For more information, refer to "The Outside of the Foot/Ankle" on page 19.

THE CALF

The calf is the biggest and most powerful muscle in the lower leg. Not only does it supply a strong force every time you take a step, but it is also active even when you think it may not be. For instance, when you're sitting in a chair, if you are pressing the ball of your foot into the ground, your calf is on and active (you might be doing this right now). Because of the constant activity of the calf, it can be a common source of pain and discomfort.

In the calf you have two main muscles: the gastrocnemius and the soleus. The much larger gastrocnemius is what you think of when you think of "calf muscles," while the slightly smaller soleus lies underneath the gastrocnemius. Since these muscles work in tandem, either can be responsible for any tightness you may feel in the calf area. They both attach to the back of the heel via the Achilles tendon, and if you're feeling discomfort mostly in that Achilles tendon, you can go back to the "Achilles Tendinitis/Tendinosis" section on page 29, where that type of pain is outlined.

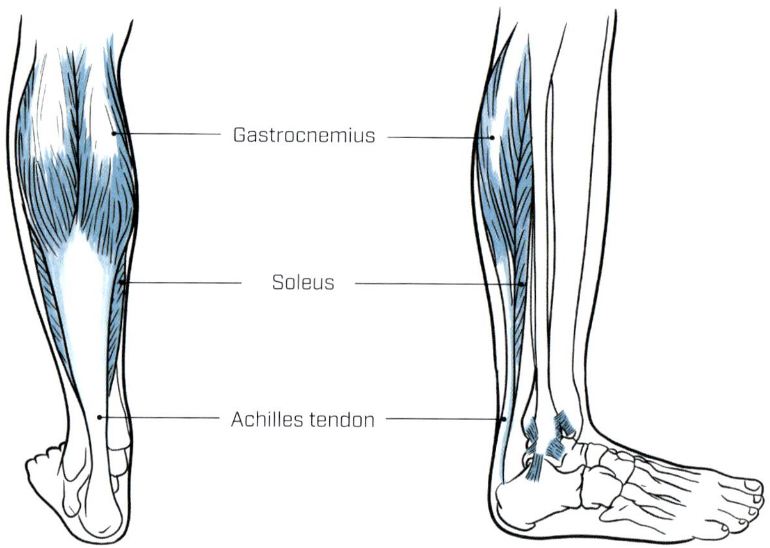

Tightness and pain in the calf tends to be at its worst after long periods of inactivity, such as when standing up first thing in the morning, or after having been seated for a couple of hours. As you continue to move and walk around and your circulation improves, you may find that the tightness starts to go down.

If that's the case, then the tightness and discomfort will respond very well to the stretches and self-massage techniques outlined at the end of this section. Start with the gentle massage techniques (see page 38), and then follow the instructions for both the gastrocnemius and soleus stretches (see pages 39 and 40). As your symptoms improve, it is important to start doing the strengthening exercises to build up control and resilience in the muscle and prevent the tightness from returning.

If you feel like no change is made in your symptoms with the self-massage and stretching and also feel like your discomfort is more of a burning or tingling pain, then you may be experiencing nerve pain related to your lower back. However, there are other conditions that can cause pain and will not respond to stretches and exercises.

DEEP VEIN THROMBOSIS (DVT)

A DVT is a blood clot most commonly found in the calf. DVTs generally develop after long periods of inactivity and can pop up after resting following surgery or sickness, or even after a long-haul flight. When you have a DVT, the pain is localized to a fairly small area in the calf. It will likely be visibly swollen and red and warm to the touch and should feel different than just a "tight muscle." It will also not respond to stretches and exercises and most often remains painful not matter what you do to it.

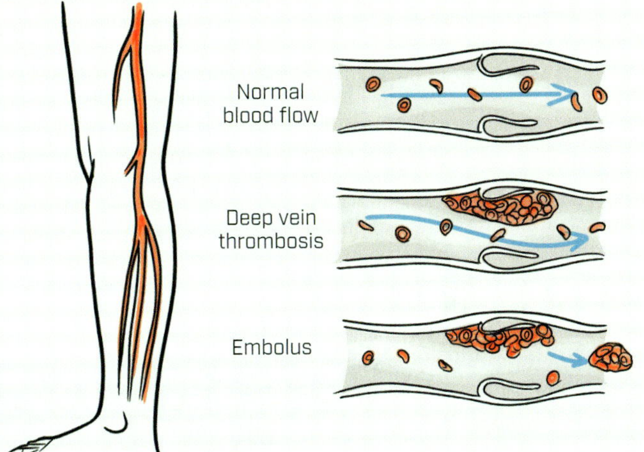

If you suspect that you have a DVT, it is important to seek immediate medical care. A professional will be able to confirm the DVT by doing an ultrasound and will administer blood thinners. It is critical that you receive this care ASAP to prevent the DVT from migrating elsewhere in the body where it can have potentially life-threatening effects.

OTHER DIAGNOSES

There is a long list of other diagnoses that can cause pain in the calf and lower leg that won't necessarily respond to stretches and exercise. As a rule, if you are experiencing symptoms that seem to be present no matter what you try to do for them, it is a good idea to seek medical attention. Almost all of the things that I outline in this book should respond within four to seven days of beginning the stretches and exercises. If you find that is not the case, it is a good idea to get medical attention sooner rather than later to prevent any serious life-altering effects.

SELF-MASSAGE TECHNIQUES & MOBILITY, FLEXIBILITY, AND STRENGTHENING MOVEMENTS FOR THE FOOT, ANKLE, AND LOWER LEG

SELF-MASSAGE

TIPS: When massaging yourself, always start gently, and make sure that your symptoms are reduced or feel about the same when you are done. If you finish the self-massage andyour symptoms have increased or you feel sore or bruised, you were likely using too much pressure. It's a good idea not to exceed five minutes per muscle group.

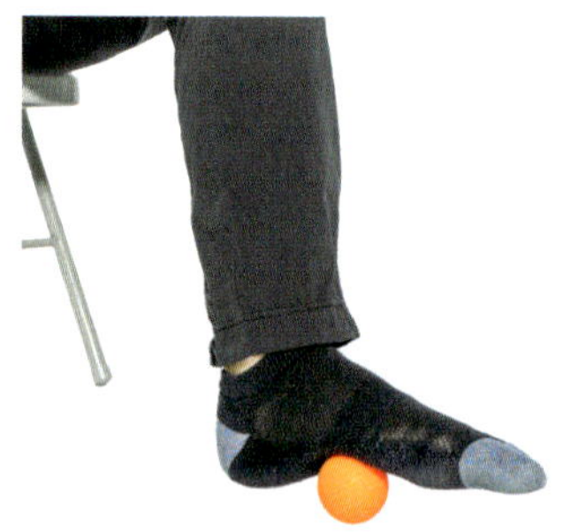

TECHNIQUE 1: ROLL OUT THE BOTTOM OF THE FOOT WITH A LACROSSE BALL

Sitting in a chair, rest your foot on a lacrosse ball. Gently move your foot over the ball as you search for tight areas. Once you find a spot that feels like a "tight" muscle, gently roll over that spot until your symptoms start to decrease. Do this for three to five minutes, and be sure to stay away from the heel and bony areas and stay mostly over the muscular areas in the arch.

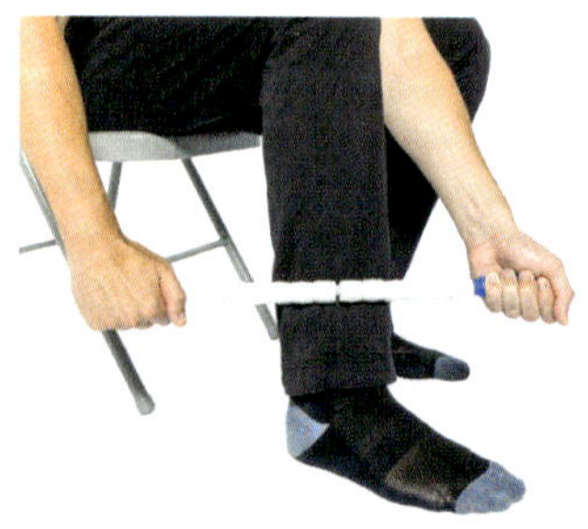

TECHNIQUE 2: GENTLE ROLLING OF THE CALF AND SHIN MUSCLES WITH A PRODUCT SIMILAR TO "THE STICK™," WHICH IS A FLEXIBLE SELF-MASSAGE TOOL

Sitting in a chair, use the stick to gently roll over muscular areas where you are experiencing tightness. Find "tight" spots and use a gentle pressure, going over the area until your symptoms start to decrease. Do this for only three to five minutes per muscle group.

TECHNIQUE 3: SELF-MASSAGE TO THE TIBIALIS POSTERIOR AND FIBULARIS LONGUS

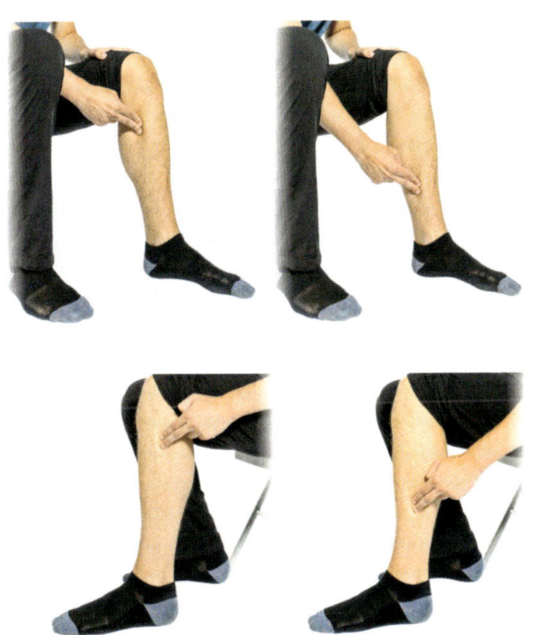

Sitting in a chair, liberally apply a lubrication agent to the area you want to massage (my favorite is cocoa butter). If massaging the tibialis posterior on the inside of the shin, use a gentle pressure with your thumb. As you get lower toward the ankle, you will reach the FHL mentioned in "The Big Toe" (page 13), which is also an effective muscle to work. If massaging the fibularis muscle group on the outside of the lower leg, use your first three fingers. In both cases, use a gentle pressure to work your way along the length of the muscle for three to five minutes, or until your symptoms start to reduce.

STRETCHES

TIPS: Keep the stretches gentle to avoid the feeling of overstretching or "pulling on the end of a tight string." Once you feel a gentle stretch, hold for twenty to twenty-five seconds and repeat three times while taking a break in between. Always make sure that you are feeling the stretch in the muscle you are targeting; if you aren't, make a slight adjustment until you do. If you respond well to these stretches, feel free to do them multiple times per day.

GASTROCNEMIUS STRETCH (2 VERSIONS)

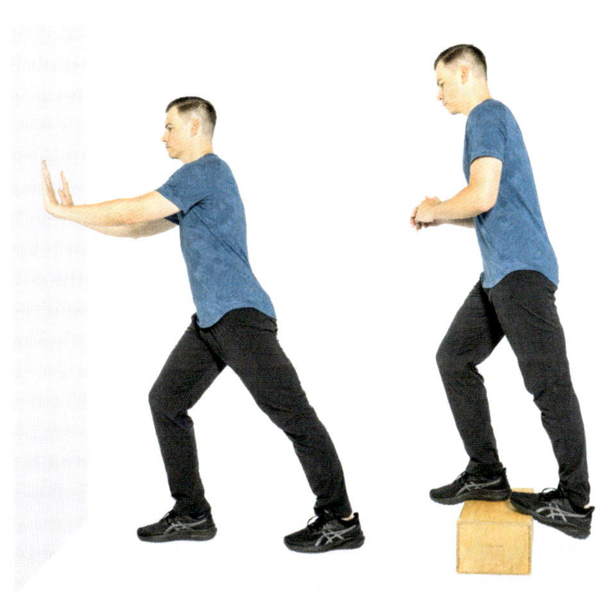

1. Standing in front of a wall, place the leg you intend to stretch in back, and keep that heel glued to the floor and the back knee locked straight. Lean toward the wall until you feel a gentle stretch in the calf of the back leg, using the wall to support you as needed.
2. Using something like a stair or curb, put the front half of your foot on the step and drop your heel to the ground while keeping your knee straight. Stop when you feel a gentle stretch in your calf.

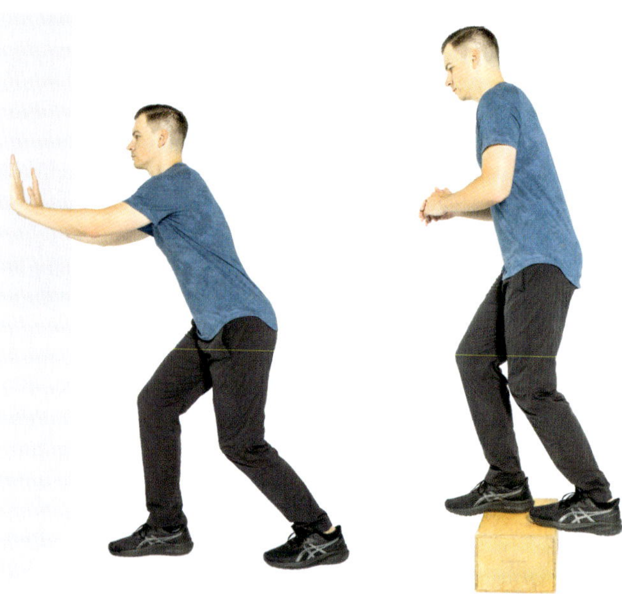

SOLEUS STRETCH (2 VERSIONS)

1. Follow the steps for the gastrocnemius stretch, but once you feel a very small stretch in your calf, bend the back knee until you feel the stretch lower toward the Achilles tendon. Hold the stretch, but be sure to keep it gentle, as this one is easier to overdo.
2. Follow the steps for the gastrocnemius stretch, but once you feel a slight stretch in your calf, bend the knee until you feel the stretch lower in the leg toward the Achilles tendon.

EXERCISES

TIPS: Try to build up to the point where you can do all of these exercises for three sets of ten repetitions with no increase in symptoms. The "sweet spot" is where you are doing these exercises at a level that feels difficult and creates muscle fatigue without an increase in symptoms or irritation. And most importantly, when in doubt, go *slower*. There really is no such thing as doing an exercise too "slow," but the faster you move, the more your form will break down, and the less likely it is that you are working the muscle group you're intending to work. Before doing any of the exercises, start with the two warm-ups.

WARM-UPS

ANKLE PUMPS

Sit with your legs straight out in front of you and bring your toes as far toward your face as you can. Then point your toes as far away from your face as you can, holding for half a second at each end. Repeat for three sets, or as many as you feel are necessary.

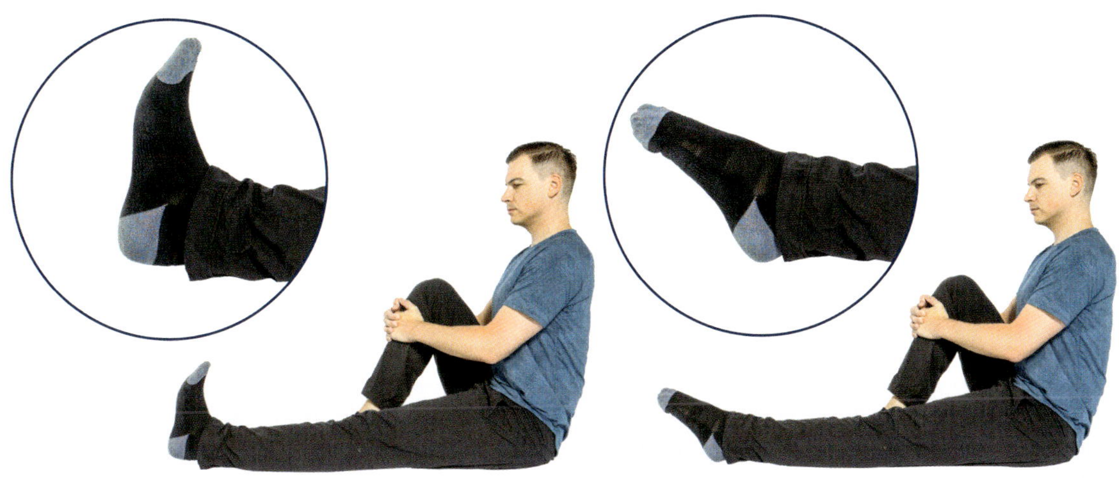

ANKLE ALPHABET

Sit with one leg straight out in front of you and draw out the alphabet with your toe as large as you can. With each letter, try to reach the end ranges of motion that you have available in the ankle. Be sure to keep the leg locked straight to ensure that all of the movement is coming from the ankle. Repeat once with uppercase letters and once with lowercase letters on each leg.

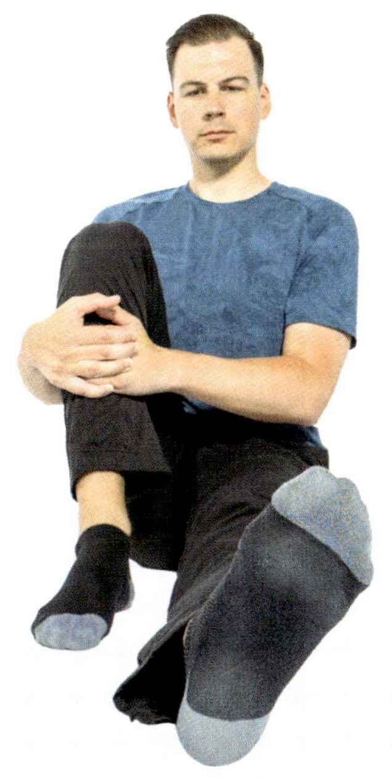

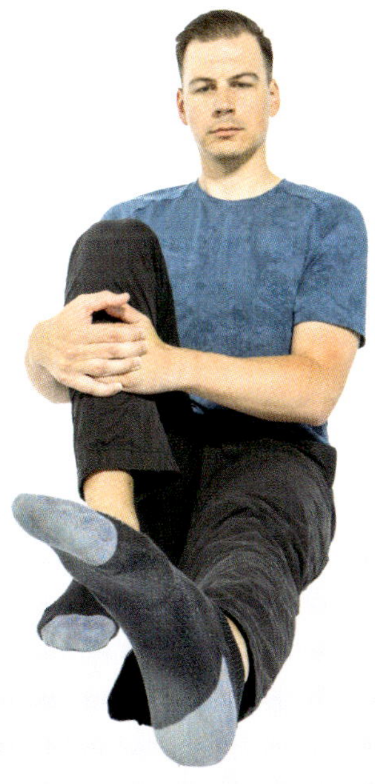

STRENGTHENING EXERCISES

ECCENTRIC HEEL RAISES

Using a chair, table, or countertop for balance if needed, rise up on your toes on both feet as high as you can go. At the top, transfer all of your weight to one side, lifting the opposite foot off the ground. From there, slowly lower your heel back to the ground on just that side. Repeat for three sets on each leg. As this exercise becomes easier, try to remove the support and get to the point where you can go up and down on just one leg.

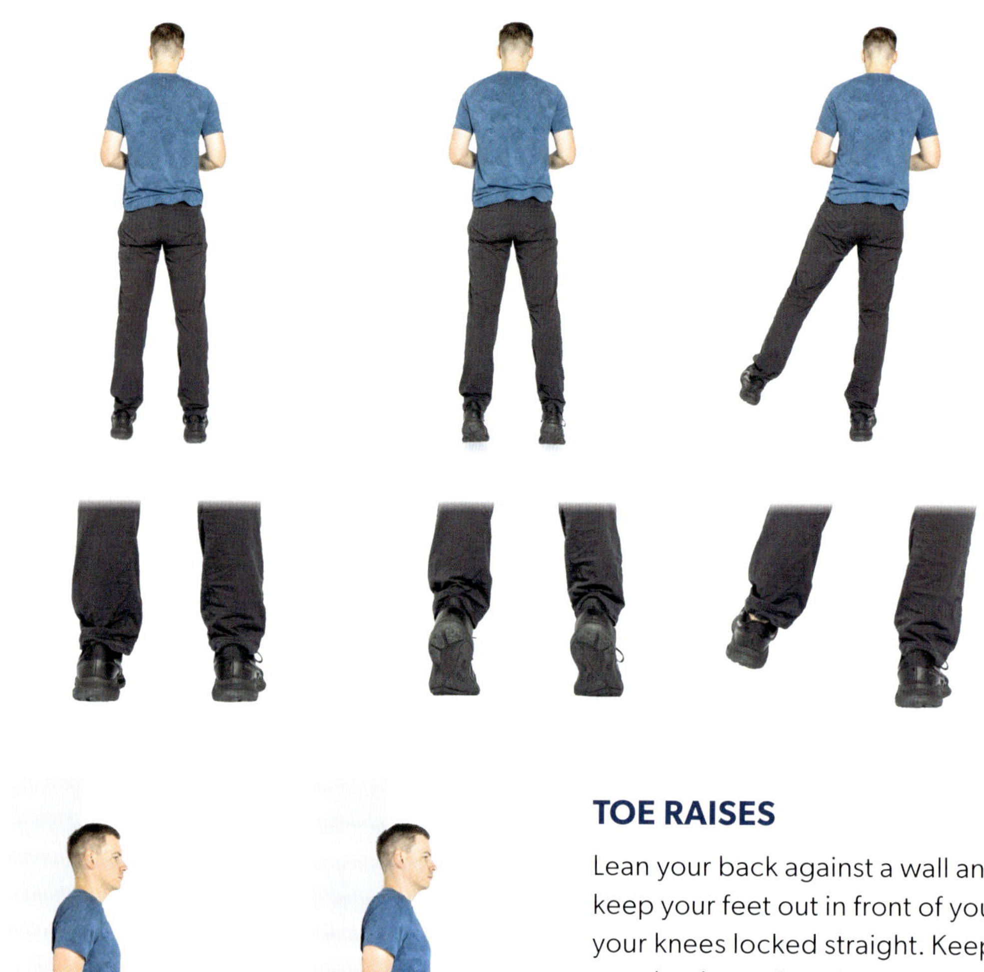

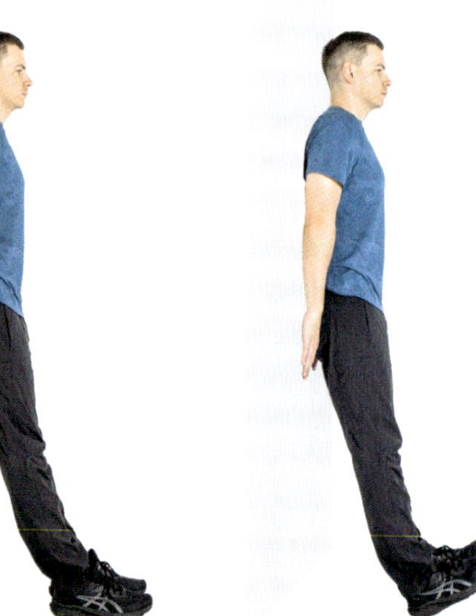

TOE RAISES

Lean your back against a wall and keep your feet out in front of you with your knees locked straight. Keeping your heels stuck to the ground, raise your toes as high as you can. You should feel a big burn in the muscles on the fronts of your shins.

BANDED ANKLE INVERSION

Sitting with your legs out in front of you, cross one leg over the other. Wrap the band around the foot of the straight leg and loop the band around the other foot. In this position, start with the foot as far out as you can and then pull it in as much as you can against the resistance of the band. Be sure to keep the leg locked straight to ensure that all of the movement is coming from the ankle.

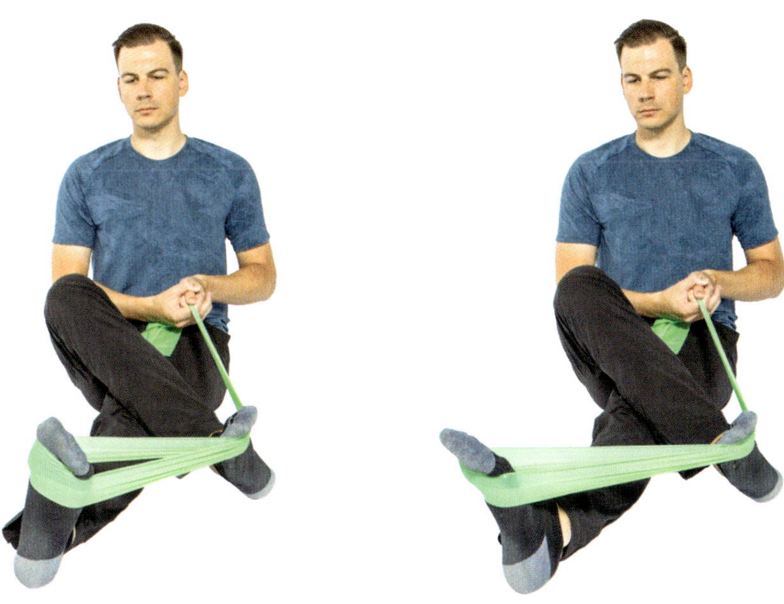

BANDED ANKLE EVERSION

Sitting with both legs out in front of you, wrap the band around the foot you want to work and loop the band around the other foot. Start with pointing the working foot in as far as you can, and then point it out as much as you can against the resistance of the band. Be sure to keep the leg locked straight to ensure that all of the movement is coming from the ankle.

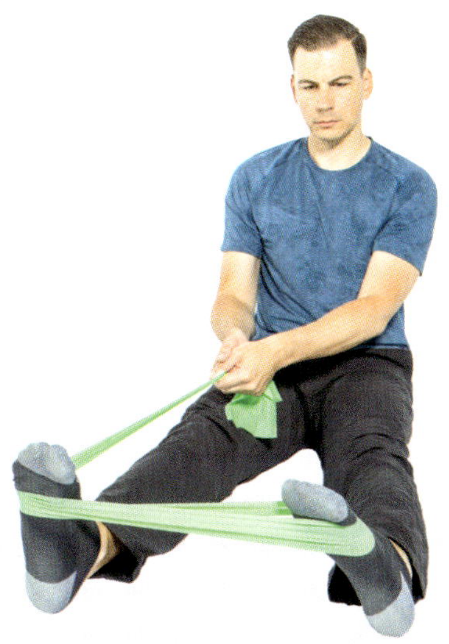

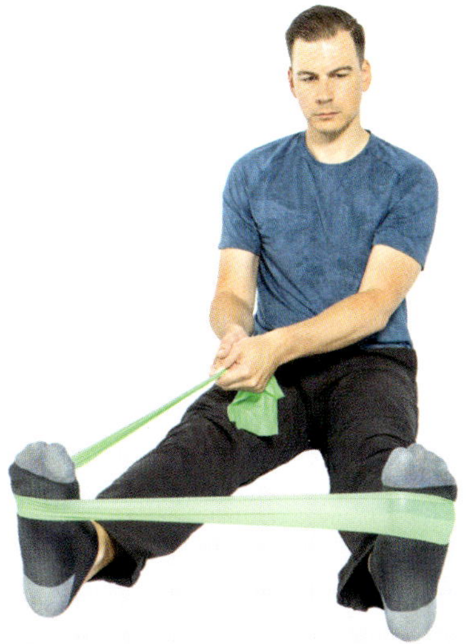

TOE YOGA

Sitting in a chair, raise just your big toe, keeping your other toes on the ground. Then try to raise the other four toes while keeping your big toe on the ground. Repeat for two sets of ten. As you become more comfortable with toe yoga, you can try other movements, like moving your big toe out to the side and then back in. Or raising all of your toes and touching them back to the ground one by one. As you challenge your toes in fun and interesting ways, it won't be long before the strength and coordination you're building really start to make a difference.

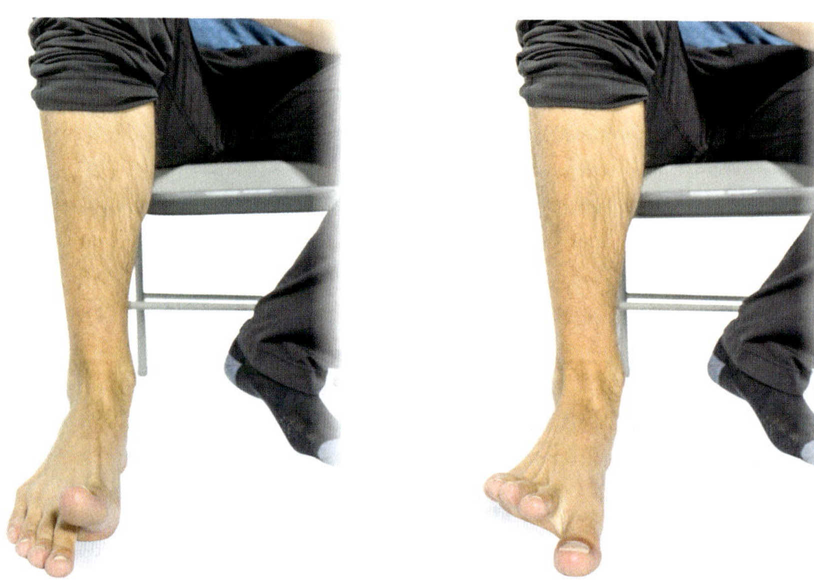

SHORT FOOT

Sitting in a chair, keep your heel and the ball of your foot on the ground as you try to "scrunch" up the arch of your foot. If you're doing it right, your foot will shorten, hence the name of the exercise. Try to keep your toes completely relaxed while doing this exercise.

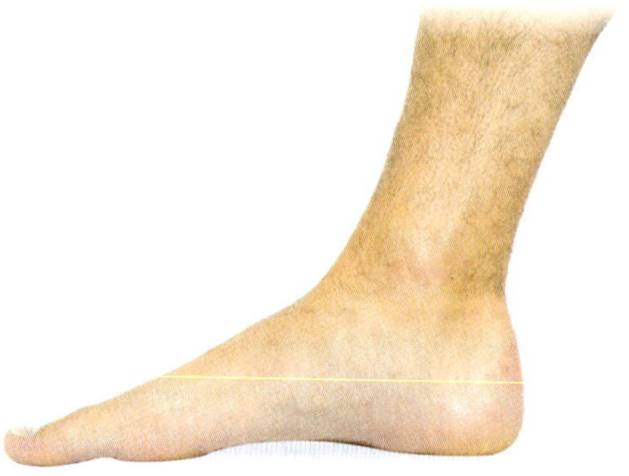

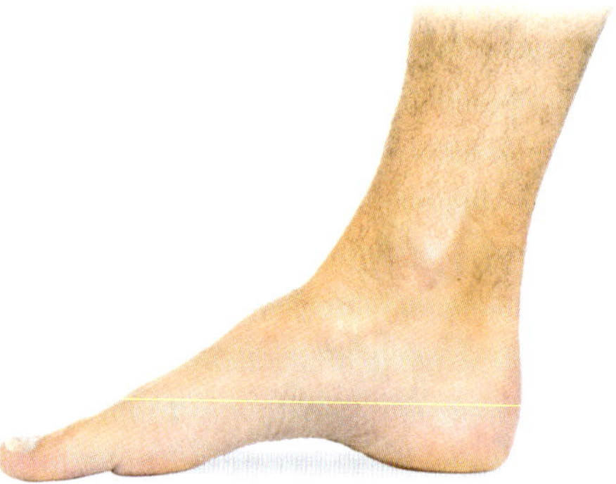

SECTION 2

THE KNEE, THE THIGH, AND THE HIP

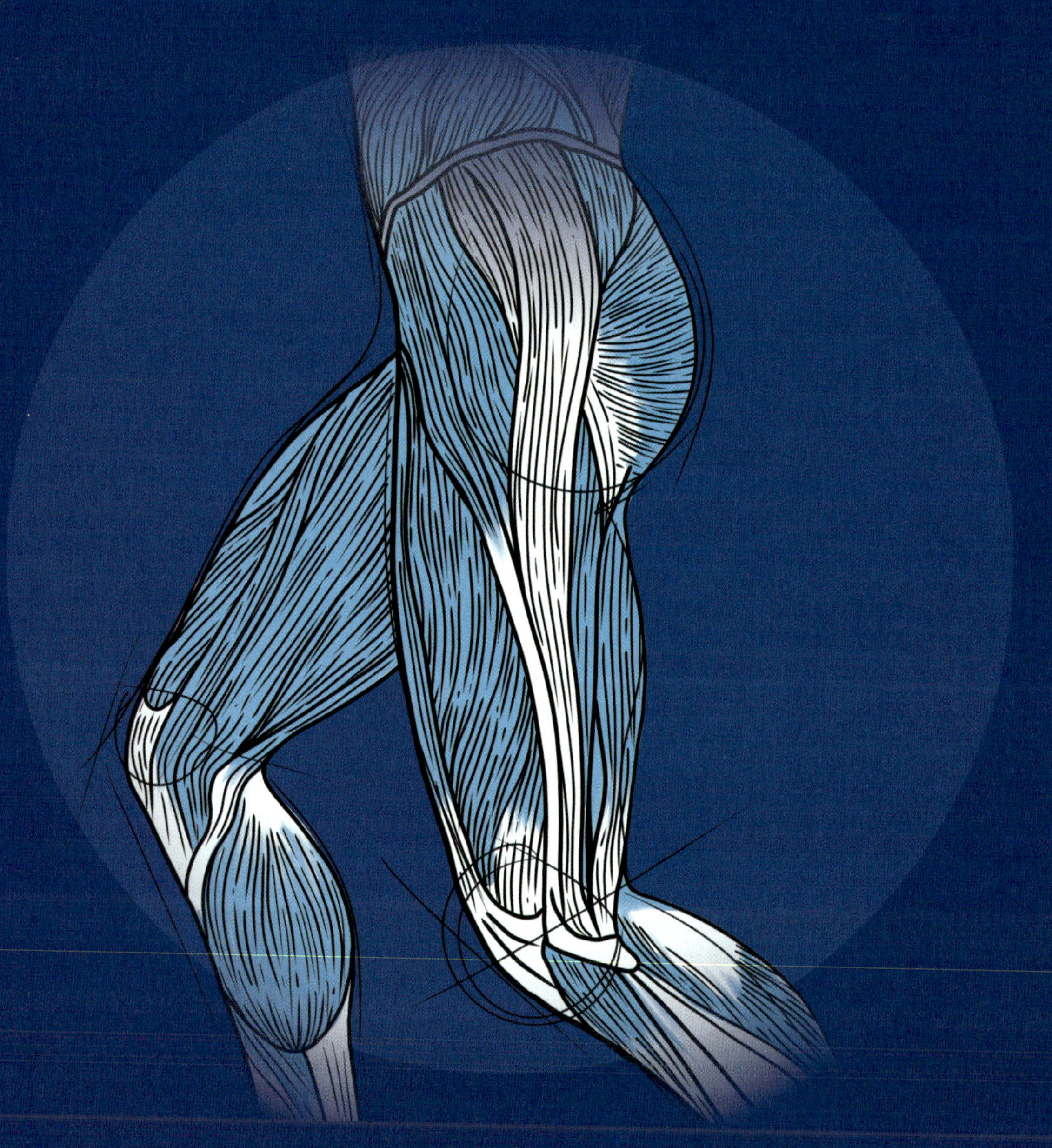

The knee is one of the most commonly injured parts of the body for a couple of reasons. The first is that it is heavily influenced by the hip. In fact, it can be argued that no other joint is as heavily influenced by another. The knee itself only moves in two directions: It can bend, and it can straighten. Anytime the knee rotates or "falls" in or out, that motion is being controlled by the hip. That is why, when looking through the sections on the inside and outside of the knee, almost all of the exercises are hip exercises.

Valgus vs. Varus Knee Alignments

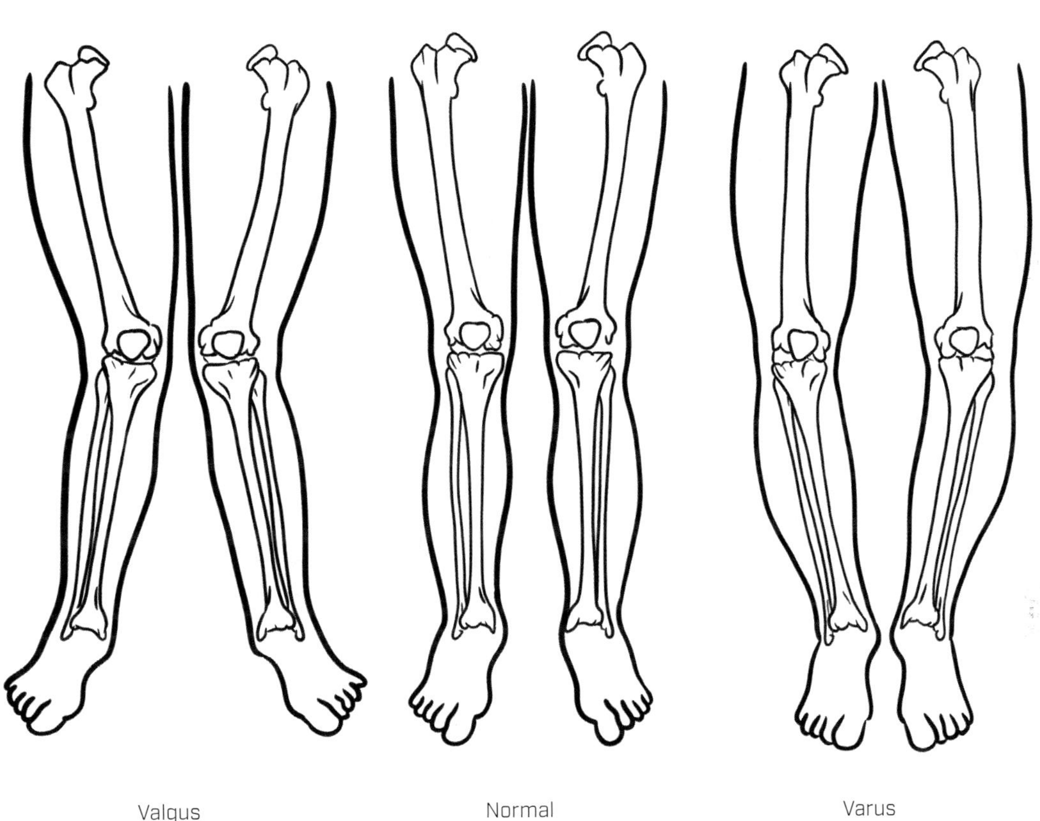

Valgus Normal Varus

Second, the major muscles that operate the knee, the quads and the hamstrings, originate extremely far away from the knee joint itself. There is no other joint in the body where the main movers start so far from that joint. Imagine trying to control a ball at the end of a string; the longer the string is, the harder of a time you'll have. And that is the struggle that the quads and hamstrings are under to bend and straighten the knee.

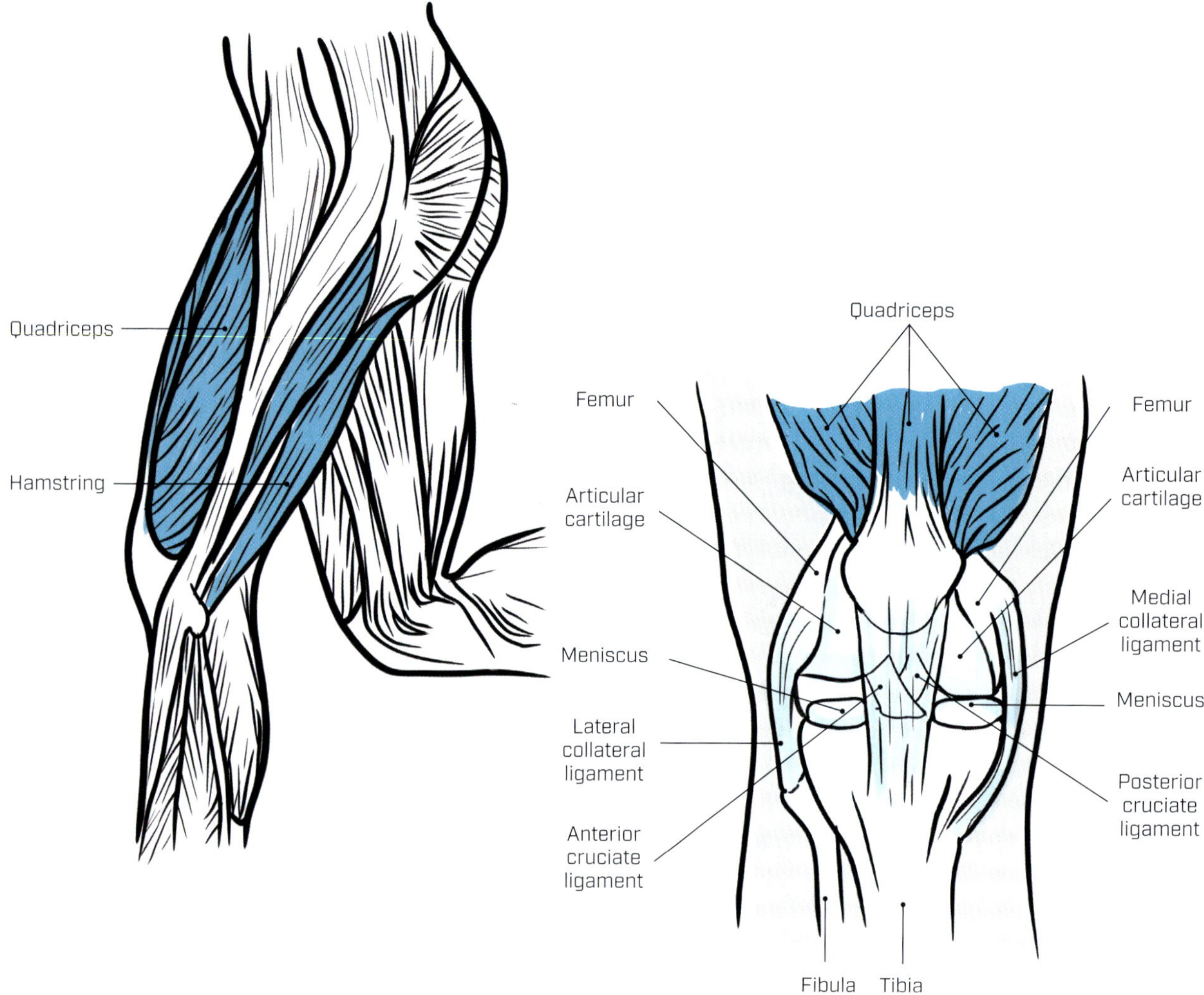

Finally, there is a lot of *stuff* (not a real anatomical term) in the knee. You have two menisci, one on the outside and one on the inside, that can be thought of as pillows of fibrocartilage that help provide cushioning. You have an anterior cruciate ligament (ACL, aka every athlete's nightmare) and a posterior cruciate ligament (PCL) that exist inside the knee joint and limit how far the tibia (shin bone) and femur (thigh bone) can slide forward and backward on each other. And you also have a medial collateral ligament (MCL) protecting the inner part of the joint and a lateral collateral ligament (LCL) protecting the outer part of the joint. That's a lot of *stuff*! And the more *stuff* that is present in a joint, the more that can go wrong.

Because of all this, the knee has kept me very busy over the years, and posts on knee pain are always my highest performers on social media. While the knee itself is a fairly simple joint, all of the factors that can create pain in the area are quite complex, which is why this is one of the longest sections in the book.

QUICK ASIDE

Before we get started with the front of the knee, let's quickly go over traumatic ACL and meniscus tears. Traumatic tears of the ACL and the meniscus most often occur when the foot is planted on the ground and the rest of the body makes a twisting movement.

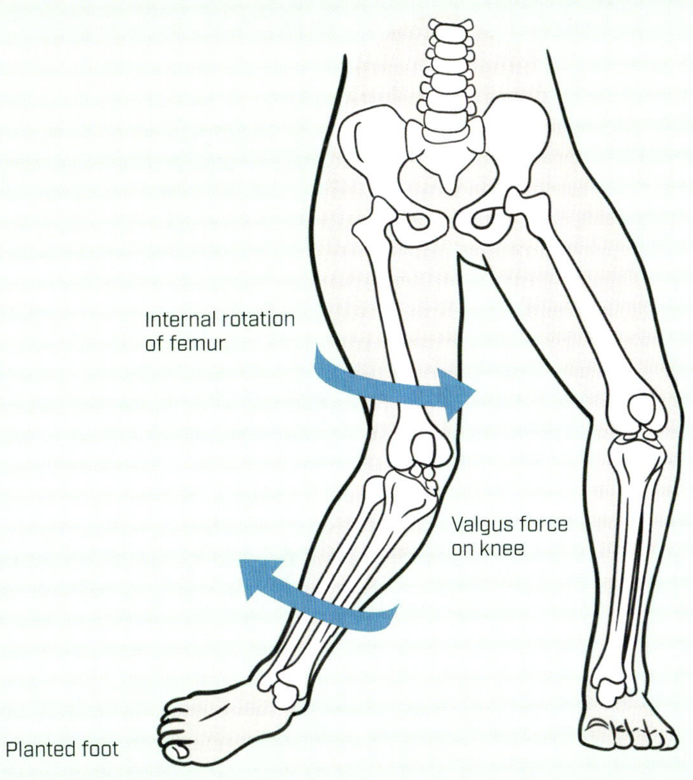

When this happens, you may hear or feel a pop (the sound of the tear taking place), and you will feel immediate pain and fall to the ground with an overwhelming sense of dread. The knee will then most often swell up (sometimes swelling will be minimal) and will sometimes bruise.

If this sounds like something you did, it is best to seek out an orthopedic MD for imaging and an official diagnosis. Even if your knee feels a lot better when the swelling finally goes down, there is still a good chance that a tear took place somewhere.

Some people with a torn ACL are able to move in a straight line just fine and feel little to no discomfort. Until, that is, they have to twist or rotate on that knee. In which case they will still feel very unstable and possibly be in pain.

So, if you can't twist on your newly injured knee, please go see an MD.

The Structures of the Front of the Knee

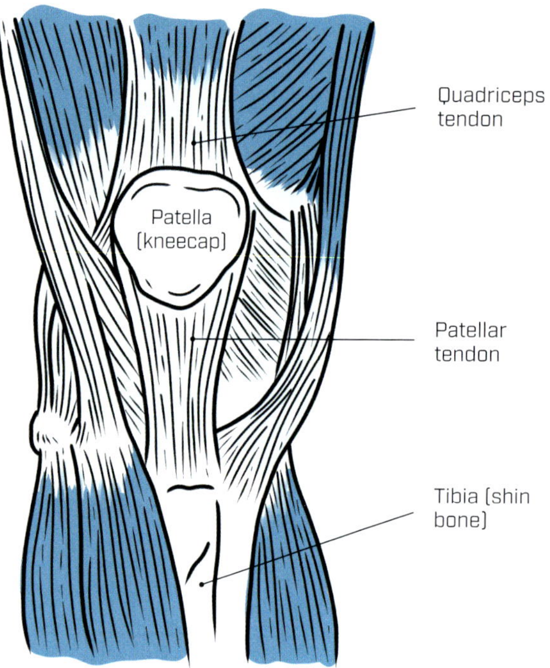

THE FRONT OF THE KNEE

In the front of the knee, you have a few major structures: the quadriceps tendon, which is where the quadriceps muscle group attaches to the patella (kneecap); the patella itself; and the patellar ligament (commonly called the patellar tendon). Note that "tendon" isn't anatomically accurate in this case, but it is still the more popular term for some reason and the term I will use throughout this section. The patellar tendon is how the patella attaches to the tibia. Anything that is causing pain in the front of the knee likely has something to do with these structures.

Anatomically speaking, a "tendon" is where muscle attaches to bone, and a "ligament" is a structure that connects bone to bone. This is the case everywhere in the body, but for some reason the patellar ligament, which connects the patella (kneecap) to the tibia (shin bone), gets called the "patellar tendon." Nobody knows how or why this happened, but it is now so commonly used that it is just accepted. Ultimately, it's not super important; it just grinds my gears enough to dedicate a few words to it.

RUNNER'S KNEE / JUMPER'S KNEE / PATELLAR TENDINITIS / PATELLAR TENDINOPATHY

All of these names are commonly used to describe one main thing: overuse and tightness in the quadriceps muscles leading to pain in the patellar tendon (ligament). It is known as both "runner's" and "jumper's" knee since that is when the pain can be felt the most. This pain is also felt when doing things like going down the stairs or bending down to tie your shoes. There may be some swelling in the area, and you may also feel an increase in pain and tightness in the quad and in the tendon when trying to bend your knee as far as it will go. If you let this pain continue without addressing it, it will slowly increase and get to the point to where it is constantly painful, and you no longer feel that you can run, jump, or tie your shoes.

Since this issue is coming from the quadriceps, the best place to start to reduce symptoms is exactly there. Start with the quad self-massage and stretches outlined on page 84 and page 86, respectively. You may also feel relief by using something like a heat pack over the quad. As blood flow and flexibility start to increase in the quad, symptoms will reduce because there is less tension in the chain and less pulling will take place at the patellar tendon.

As symptoms ease, it's a good idea to start doing all of the exercises at the end of this section, but one in particular is heavily backed by research to get this pain to go away for good. That exercise is the long arc quad isometric hold (it's a bit of a mouthful, I know; see page 88). In order to get the full effect from these exercises, you are going to want to hold the exercise for forty-five seconds and repeat for a set of ten. Alternatively, you can hold for twenty-two seconds and repeat twenty times, since the research suggests that all that matters is the total time under tension.

Finally, you should work up to the point where you can do the step-down exercise (see page 89) with no irritation of your symptoms. Ideally, when doing any of these exercises, you should feel muscle fatigue in the quad but no increase in pain. The step-down is what will start to make things like running and going down the stairs a lot more stable and comfortable.

A good target would be to complete these exercises every other day, as long as no symptoms are aggravated and muscle soreness doesn't build up too much.

OSGOOD-SCHLATTER DISEASE

Osgood-Schlatter's presentation is extremely similar to runner's/jumper's knee, but the cause is different. Osgood-Schlatter is most common in adolescents going through a growth spurt because bones grow faster than muscles and tendons. This leads to a lot of stress and strain where the patellar tendon (ligament) attaches at the tibia. If there is enough tension for long enough, the attachment site can get swollen, and the body may even create a bony bump where the irritation is.

As with runner's/jumper's knee, the best place to start to reduce symptoms is with self-massage techniques over the quadriceps to try to reduce the tension. It is also a good idea to incorporate some stretching to increase flexibility of the quad. Make sure you feel the stretch in the muscle itself and keep it gentle. If you are only feeling more tension and pain at the site of irritation, then it is a good idea to stick to self-massage for a while.

Ultimately, since this diagnosis is tied to growing, most people just have to wait until their growth spurt has ended for symptoms to fully subside. Sometimes the bump that occurred from the irritation never goes away, although it should become less sensitive. Once fully grown, it is a good idea to follow the quad-centric techniques starting on page 83 to ensure a strong, healthy, and flexible muscle.

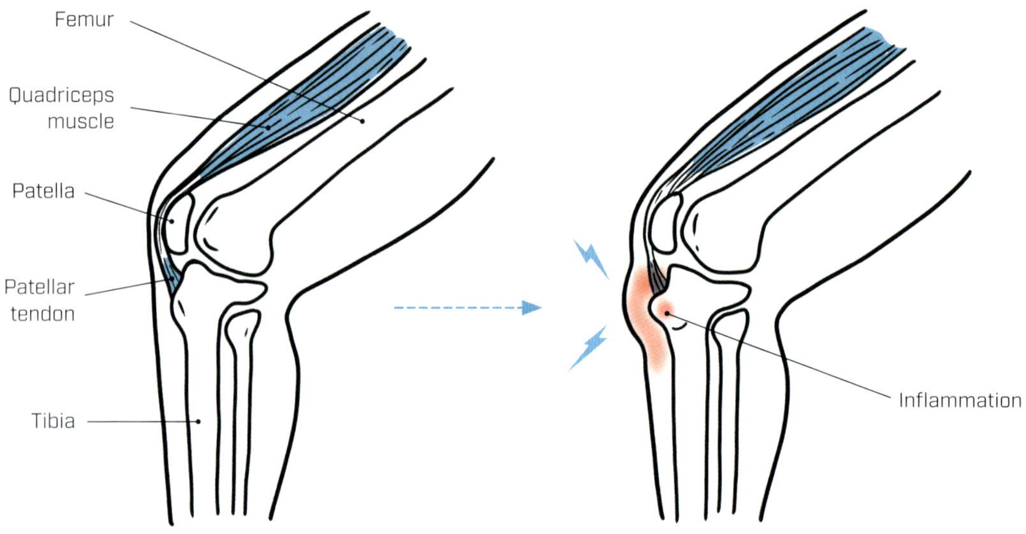

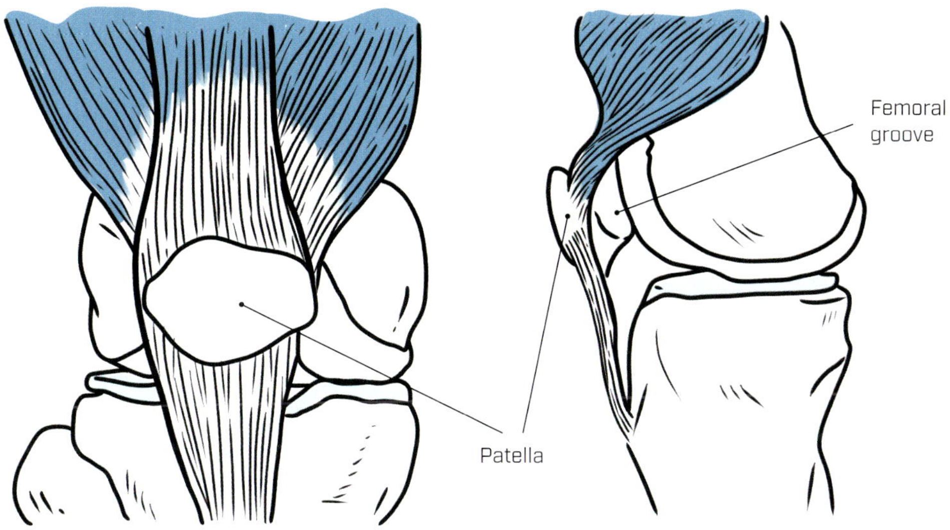

PATELLOFEMORAL PAIN SYNDROME

Patellofemoral pain syndrome (PFPS) has become a diagnosis used to describe almost every possible source of pain that is felt on the patella (kneecap) itself. In practice, PFPS is used very broadly and can mean a lot of different things to a lot of different practitioners. In this book, I am using PFPS to describe pain that exists on either the inside or the outside of the patella.

If you experience pain on the outside edges of the patella, it likely means that you are having an issue with how well the patella is tracking while the knee is bending and straightening. If the patella doesn't stay perfectly in its groove, it can become irritated as it rides up against the edge of the groove.

As with the two previous diagnoses, this can have something to do with the quadriceps, since that is the only muscle group that directly attaches to the patella. So, it is a good idea to address the quad with self-massage, flexibility, and strengthening techniques. But this issue likely has more to do with the strength and control of the hips.

Biomechanically, the knee joint really only flexes and extends; most of the rotation and movement of the knee from side to side comes from the hips. And if there is weakness in the rotators of the hips, it can allow the knee to fall "out of line," and that stress can cause irritation in the sides of the patella.

If your knees cave in when going down into a squat, or if one of your knees wants to fall in or out when going up a set of stairs, then this likely relates to you. Addressing the quad will provide short-term relief, but for long-term relief, it is important to become as strong as possible into hip rotation in order to maintain stability in the knee. Those exercises can be found starting on page 84.

The Knee "Falling" In or Out

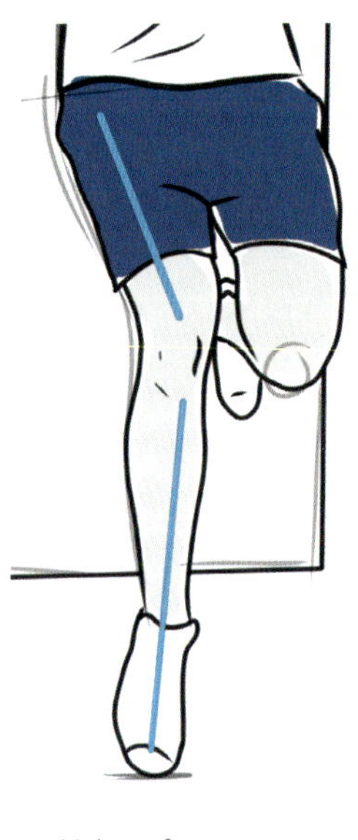

Valgus force

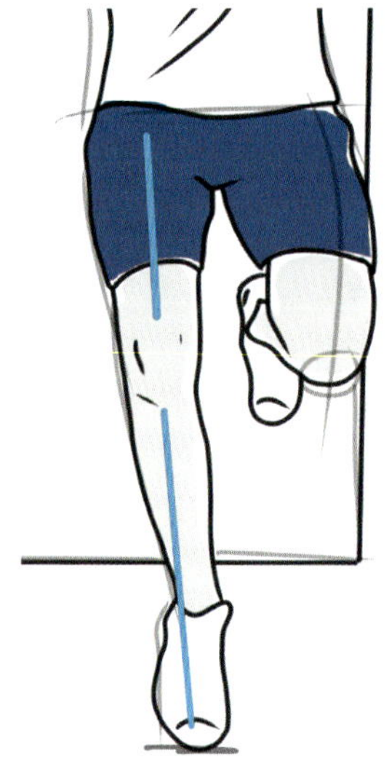

No valgus force

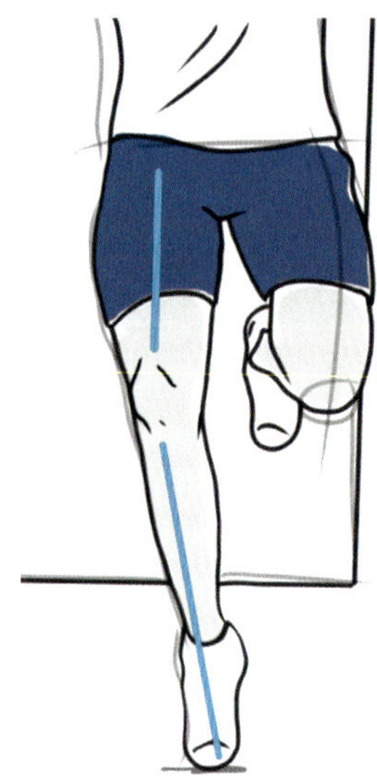

Varus force

PREPATELLAR BURSITIS

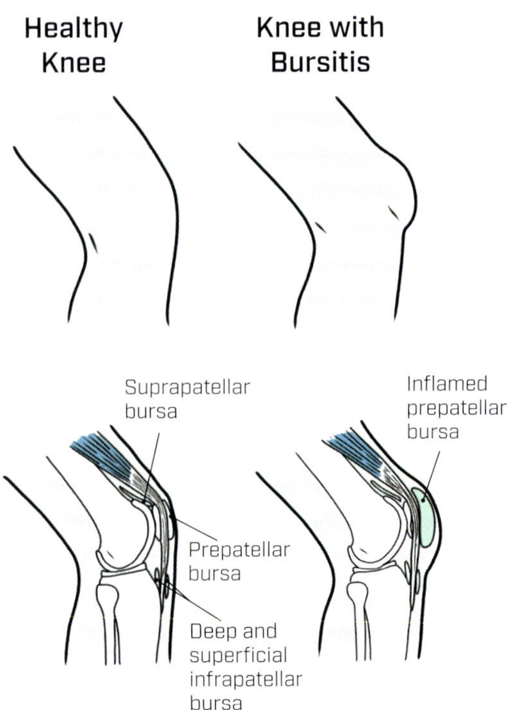

Prepatellar bursitis is when pain and swelling develops in a bursa right on the middle of the kneecap. You have bursas throughout the body; they are basically fluid-filled sacs that absorb shock and reduce friction in joints. They are necessary for movement, but when they become irritated, they can wreak havoc.

This bursa is either irritated slowly over time in people who spend a lot of time on their knees or becomes irritated all at once if someone falls directly on the knee. In some cases, there is a lot of swelling and warmth in the bursa, and it is extremely sensitive to the touch.

The best course of action is to avoid further irritation of the area by avoiding being on your knees. In most cases, the swelling will go down all by itself. If the swelling does not begin to go down even as you avoid putting any pressure on the area, it's a good idea to seek medical care to see what else can be done.

TIBIAL PLATEAU FRACTURE

A tibial plateau fracture can create pain anywhere at the top of the tibia where it meets the femur. It can occur after something like jumping down from a great height, or it can be caused by repetitive stress. Pain will greatly increase when you're on your feet for a while, and it normally feels like a deep, aching discomfort. The best thing to do when experiencing these symptoms is to see an orthopedic MD to get X-ray imaging and receive an official diagnosis. If the fracture is small, you may just need to take it easy and keep weight off the affected leg until it has a chance to heal. If the fracture is larger, the MD may suggest surgery.

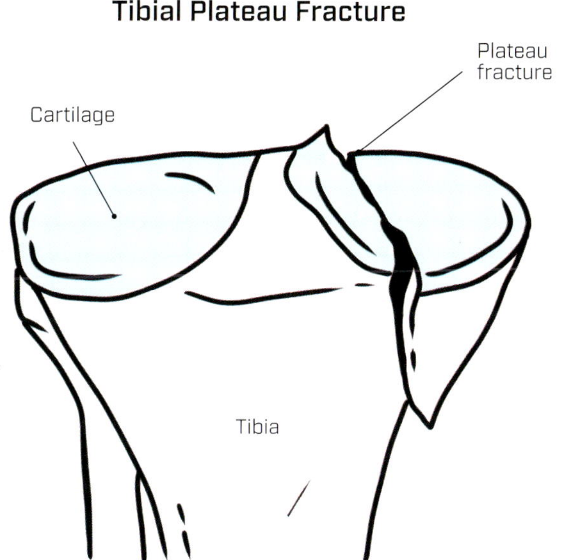

THE INSIDE AND OUTSIDE OF THE KNEE

Two diagnoses can present on one or both sides of the knee joint since the causes are present on each side. A meniscus issue is almost always on one side and not the other, but arthritis can sometimes cause pain in both sides of the joint. The other diagnoses that only present on either the inside *or* the outside of the knee are because of specific structures that are only on one side and not the other.

ARTHRITIS

Arthritis is a scary word to many people, but when you break it down, you can see it doesn't have to be the life-altering diagnosis that a lot of people make it out to be.

Arth is the Latin term for "joint," and *-itis* is Latin for "inflammation." Arthritis literally just translates to "joint inflammation." Inflammation of the joints is just as normal a sign of aging as wrinkles or grey hair. Nearly one in five adults have been officially diagnosed with some form of arthritis, and that number jumps up to nearly one in two adults over the age of sixty-five. But these are just people who have received an official diagnosis. It's estimated that the true prevalence of arthritis is much higher; it just hasn't been painful, so people have not had it officially diagnosed.

There are also studies that show that arthritis isn't necessarily linked to the pain and symptoms it is associated with. Major surveys have shown that 60 percent of people with diagnosed arthritis claim to have mild to no symptoms in the diagnosed joint, which means that just because you are showing arthritis on an X-ray image, it doesn't mean that it is the cause of your pain. That is especially the case in the knee. I have seen a lot of patients with knee pain who have arthritis that shows up on imaging but whose pain had nothing to do with that arthritis.

Arthritis in the Knee

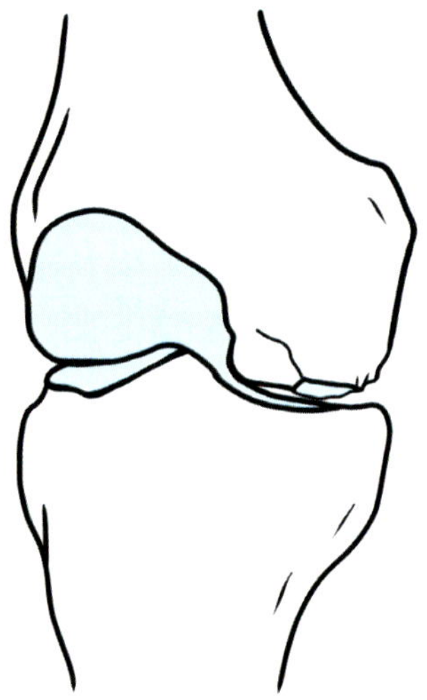

PATIENT STORY

Early in my career, I had a patient referred to me by a surgeon who was going to perform a total knee replacement in six weeks. Before the surgery, he wanted the patient to gain as much strength and range of motion as possible to make the recovery process easier. When I evaluated her, I found that she had fairly severe knee pain, but her symptoms didn't align with arthritis at all. Instead, it seemed like a textbook case of pes anserine bursitis (more on this on page 60). After just four weeks of treating the muscles associated with my diagnosis, she was pain free and canceled her surgery.

This is my favorite example of making sure that just because you may be a certain age and have a diagnosed case of something like arthritis, that doesn't mean that it is where your pain is coming from.

If your pain is from arthritis, you will likely have pain both when fully straightening the knee and when fully bending the knee. You will also likely have pain when trying to kneel or get into a deep squat. Your pain may get worse in cold and rainy weather, and your knee will feel stiff in the morning or after you have been sedentary for a while. Finally, the pain will likely get worse the longer you walk or spend time on your feet.

If your symptoms don't align with that presentation, there is a chance that your knee pain is not coming from arthritis, and you may find your answer elsewhere in this book.

If your symptoms do align with arthritis, it is still a good idea to follow the exercises and stretches at the end of this section, starting on page 83. The weaker and tighter your muscles are, the more stress is placed on your joints. Simply by gaining strength and flexibility, you can reduce the load placed on the joints, which can greatly reduce pain and inflammation. And just like in the patient story, even if you are destined for something like a total knee reconstruction, the stronger and more flexible you are before the surgery, the easier the recovery process will be. So, you have nothing to lose. Get moving!

MENISCUS TEARS

In your knee, you have two menisci: one on the inside of your knee, called the medial meniscus, and one on the outside of your knee, called the lateral meniscus. You can think of them as cushions that help to absorb the forces of walking, running, and jumping. When they are healthy, they allow the knee to glide smoothly as you straighten and bend it and provide protection when you need to plant and twist on your leg.

Medial and Lateral Menisci in the Knee

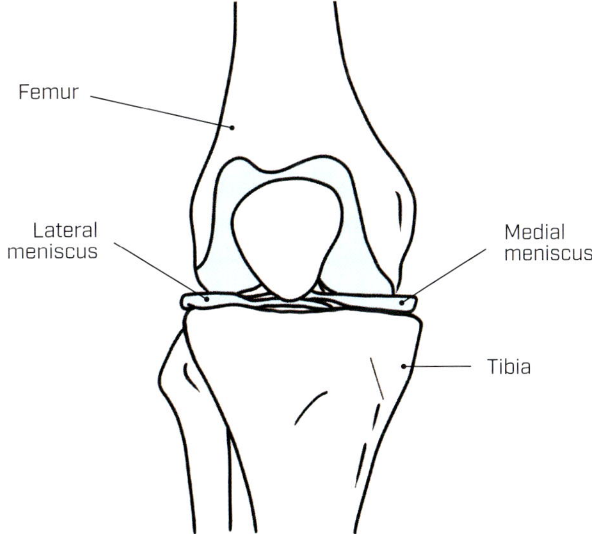

When there is a tear present in one of the menisci, there are a few hallmark signs. The first is that pain will normally increase when the knee is fully straight or fully bent. You will also likely experience a popping or clicking sensation on the side where you feel the pain every time your knee passes a certain angle. Along with this, you will likely feel very unstable trying to plant and twist on the leg where you have the pain.

This is because when there is a tear in the meniscus, a little bit of that tear flaps upward, and what once was a nice, smooth surface now has a speed bump, which is what causes the clicking and the pain with bending and straightening. The meniscus also helps provide rotational stability, so when it is compromised, planting and twisting is a nightmare.

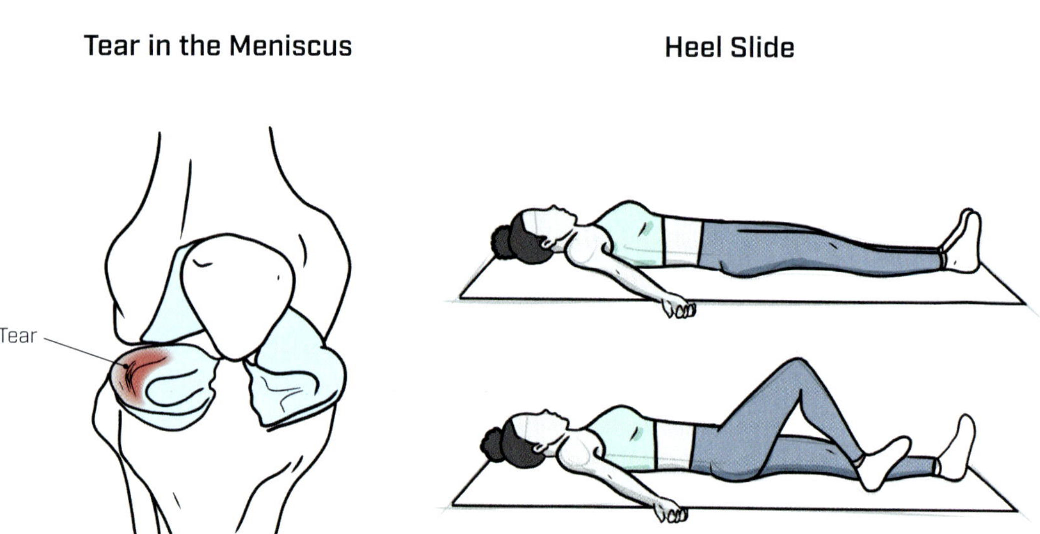

Larger tears may require surgery, but most tears in the meniscus are very small and respond extremely well to physical therapy. In PT, the first goal is to restore pain-free range of motion in the knee. The best way to start is by doing the heel slide exercise above. This exercise may be uncomfortable to start, but the more you do it, the easier and less painful the motion should become. The goal is that the repeated motion helps the tear to sort of "lie down" and prevents the tear from limiting the motion. If the tear can stay that way for a period of time, it can begin to heal and scar over in a way that is no longer painful. I normally suggest that people with a small meniscus tear do this exercise twenty to thirty times at least two or three times per day.

As the pain-free range of motion returns, it is a good idea to strengthen the entire leg with the exercises found at the end of the section. The stronger the muscles are, the less strain is placed on the joint and the meniscus.

I have seen tons of cases of small meniscus tears improve in PT, but if you have been focusing on these exercises for two to four weeks with no improvement, it may be time to see a sports or orthopedic MD.

THE INSIDE OF THE KNEE

There are three major causes of pain on the inside of the knee that I have seen in my years as a PT. The first is a tear in the medial meniscus, which is addressed above. The next is an issue with the medial collateral ligament (MCL), which is the major ligament that runs on the inside of the knee. The third is an issue with the muscles that make up the pes anserine (a collection of three separate tendons that attach to the same spot on your shin bone).

Structures of the Inside of the Knee

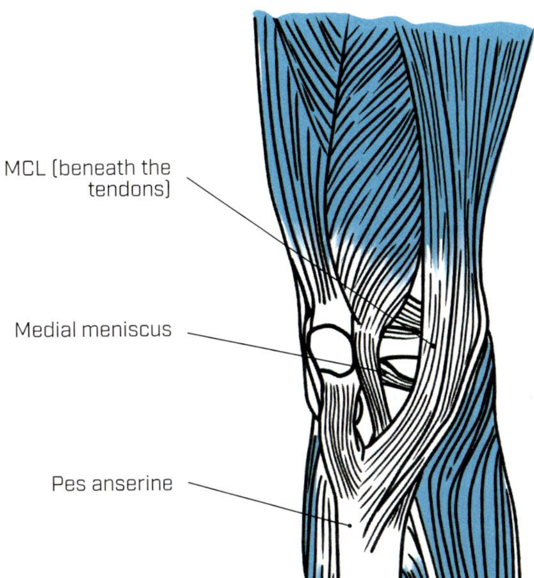

MCL TEAR / LAXITY

The medial collateral ligament (MCL) is a large ligament that provides stability to the inside of the knee, and if you hurt it, you likely know it. The most common way to injure the MCL is with a valgus blow to the knee, or a sideways blow that knocks your knee toward your other knee. (Valgus is when your knee caves inward, and varus is when your knee caves outward.)

It's hard to sustain a blow like this without knowing it. And if you did, it is likely a good idea to just go straight to a healthcare practitioner to rule out serious damage.

But it's also possible for the MCL to just be a little lax, and if you've ever been described as "knock-kneed," this may be the case for you. If the MCL is lax, then your knees will collapse inward, and if your knee falls inward, then it will put strain on the MCL and make it lax. The chicken or the egg of it all doesn't truly matter; what does matter is getting your femur into external rotation to get your knee back into a better alignment.

Improving strength and flexibility in your hips is the key to addressing any symptoms in your MCL or preventing any from developing. The stronger the external rotators of your hip are, the less likely it is that your knee will collapse inward when doing any number of things, including squats and going up and down the stairs. No matter what has compromised your MCL, the best path forward is to focus on the hip rotation exercises at the end of this section (starting on page 83) and trying your best not to allow your knee to collapse inward with challenging movements.

Valgus Force to the Knee

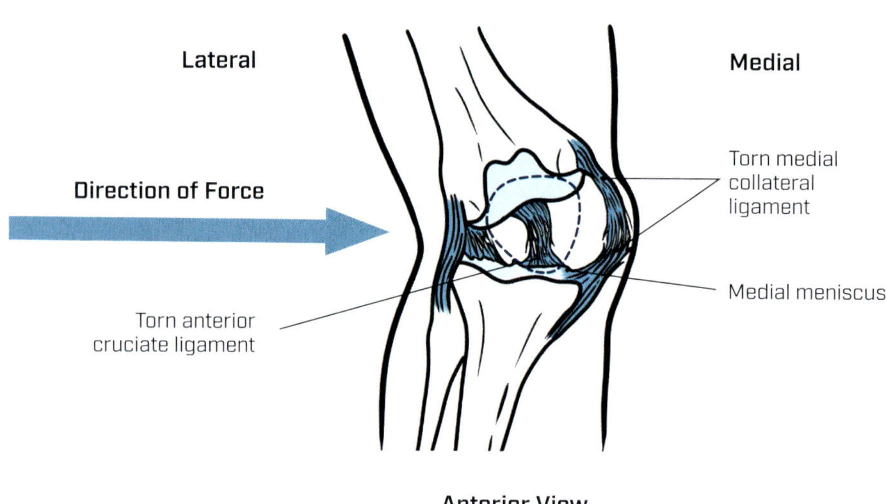

Anterior View

PES ANSERINE BURSITIS / TENDINITIS

The pes anserine is a common attachment site in the shin for three muscles in the thigh. In fact, *pes anserine* is Latin for "goose's foot," because the spot where these three muscles attach resembles the foot of a goose. And anytime you have multiple muscles attaching to the same spot on a bone, you can run into trouble. The three muscles are the semitendinosus (an inner hamstring muscle), gracilis (a groin muscle), and sartorius (the longest muscle in the body, which runs from the hip and over the quads). Each of these three muscles can be the culprit when there is pain on the inside of the knee.

Pes Anserine Attachments

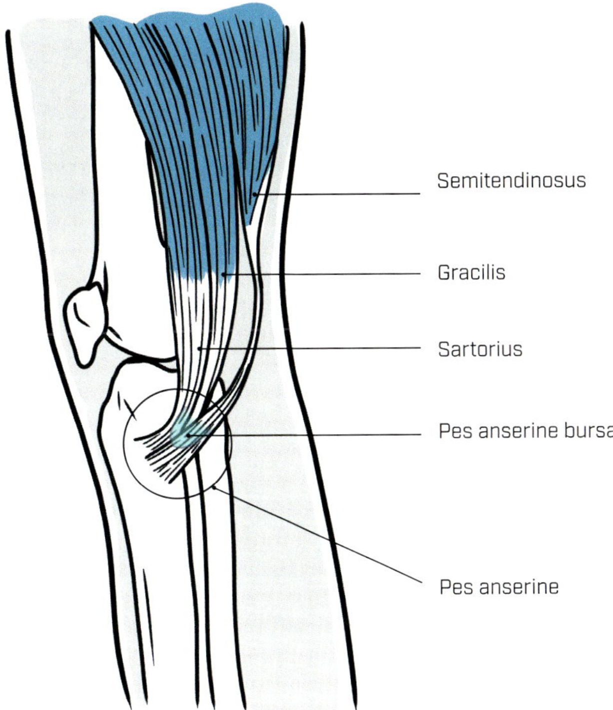

I've really only seen the sartorius be the cause of knee symptoms if you tend to frequently cross your legs when you're sitting. When you cross one leg over the other, the leg on top has the sartorius in a shortened position, and if you are in that position often enough, the sartorius can create discomfort at the pes anserine. If the knee where you're feeling the pain is on the side that you normally keep crossed over the other leg, stop crossing your legs. If you resist the urge for two weeks and all of a sudden the inside of your knee is feeling better, then you have your answer.

The gracilis and semitendinosus in the pes aserine tend to become tight and painful because of overuse. This can happen when the muscles aren't strong enough to handle whatever activity you are putting them through on a regular basis.

The best place to start is by using the self-massage and stretching techniques for both the hamstring and the groin found starting on page 85. If after a few days, you notice that the knee is feeling better, then you can also start doing the strengthening exercises for those two muscle groups. The goal is that after three to four weeks, the pain on the inside of the knee is markedly better. To keep it that way, you just have to ensure that you maintain the flexibility and strength of the groin and hamstring. And, as a general rule, it's also a good idea to do all of the knee-related exercises in this book to make sure that the entire leg is as strong and symmetrical as possible.

THE OUTSIDE OF THE KNEE

The outside of the knee is pretty similar to the inside of the knee; there are three main diagnoses that I've seen cause pain, and the anatomy is fairly similar. The first cause of pain is a meniscus tear (see page 49), the next is a lateral collateral ligament injury, and the third is from the illiotibial (IT) band, which starts much farther up the leg.

The 3 Major Structures That Can Cause Pain in the Lateral Knee

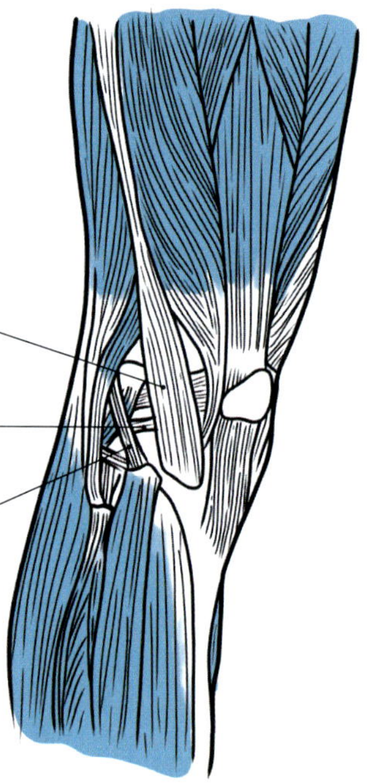

IT band

Lateral meniscus

LCL

LCL TEAR / LAXITY

The lateral collateral ligament (LCL) is much harder to injure than its counterpart on the inside of the knee, the medial collateral ligament (MCL). That's because the outside of the knee is much more stable. It's far more common to suffer an injury where the knee falls inward rather than outward. In order to sustain an injury to the LCL, you likely would need some sort of force or blow to the inside of the knee that forces the knee outward.

If you do suffer something like this, then it is a good idea to see a medical professional to rule out anything serious.

The LCL can also be a little lax. If you feel like you've always been a little bowlegged, this may be you. The less stable the ligament is on the outside of the knee, the more the knee will push outward.

To try to correct for this, you can focus on the exercises that increase strength and mobility into hip internal rotation. Being strong and mobile into hip internal rotation (see page 84) will help alleviate stress on the LCL and outside of the knee. And if you're able to use this strength and mobility to prevent the knee from falling outward, you can hopefully greatly reduce your symptoms.

ILLIOTIBIAL (IT) BAND PAIN (KNEE)

The illiotibial (IT) band is a long, broad ligament that runs along the outside of your leg and attaches on the outside of the knee. Pain at the knee caused by the IT band most often pops up after prolonged exercise such as walking, running, biking, or elliptical training. You may also feel an increase in pain on the outside of the knee every time you take your knee from slightly bent to fully straight. But the easiest way to confirm that your IT band is responsible for your discomfort is either to have someone press into the side of your thigh or to lie on a foam roller with the side of your thigh. If you find it incredibly painful, the IT band is your culprit.

The main muscular attachment of the IT band is the tensor fasciae latae (TFL), but it can also attach to the outside of the quad and hamstring as it makes its way down toward the knee. Since the IT band is not a muscle, when you're using the self-massage techniques at the end of this section on page 83, you're going to want to focus on these three muscles. Trying to massage directly over the IT band itself will mostly just create a lot of discomfort without really providing much help. Taking away tension from these three muscles using the self-massage techniques should hopefully reduce your symptoms.

The best way to create long-term change in the IT band is to focus on the exercises that work on the mobility and strength of internal hip rotation and exercises that strengthen the hip abductors. The weaker and more immobile you are in internal hip rotation, the more irritated the TFL will be. The weaker the hip abductors are, the more unsupported the TFL is.

If you're able to focus on all of that consistently for three to four weeks, you should see a huge change in the tightness and discomfort along the outside of your leg and knee.

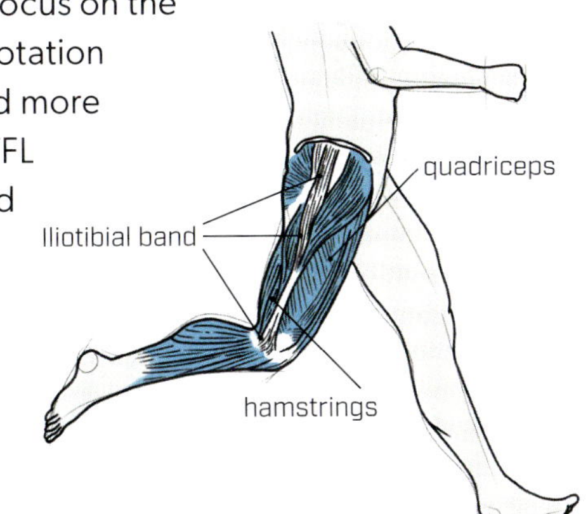

THE BACK OF THE KNEE

When pain is present in the back of the knee, it is usually due to an issue with one of the two main structures that cross the back of the knee: the hamstring and the calf. (That being said, if you do have a small meniscus tear, you may feel a pain in the back of the knee when straightening or fully bending it, so the "Meniscus Tears" section on page 49 is worth reading.)

You may also feel pain in the back of the knee if you have injured your posterior cruciate ligament (PCL). This is the ligament that runs behind its much more famous counterpart, the ACL. This pain is present mostly when kneeling or doing something

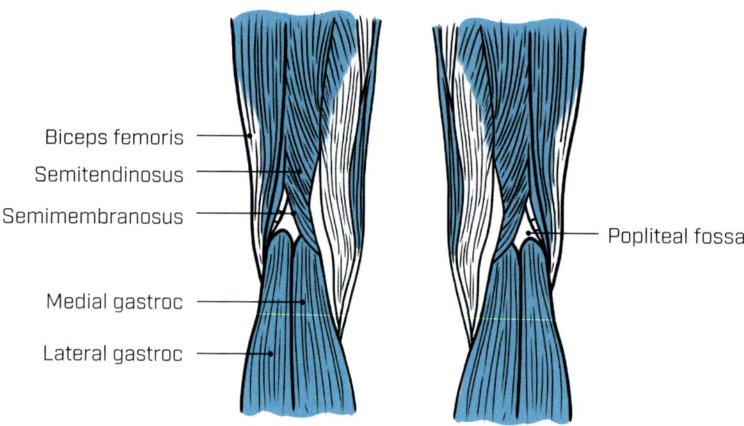

like going down a set of stairs. The most common way to hurt it is to sustain a blow to the front of the knee that pushes the knee directly backward, hyperextending it. If you suffered an injury like that and the other information in this section isn't helpful, you may have a PCL injury and should see a medical professional to rule out a serious tear.

But for the most part, pain that has been present for a while in the back of the knee where there was no major, traumatic injury almost always ties back to the hamstring and the calf.

HAMSTRING TENDINITIS/ TENDINOSIS

The hamstring is a group of three muscles that run down the back of your leg. On the inside, you have the semitendinosus and the semimembranosus, and on the outside, you have the biceps femoris.

When the knee is bent, the hamstring is in a shortened position. Considering how many people spend most of the day seated in a chair or on a couch, it makes sense that so many people feel tightness in their hamstrings. It also makes sense that hamstring tightness is most often felt when getting up after spending a long period of time sitting. Sometimes that discomfort is felt right over the muscle, but in a lot of cases, the pain presents where the hamstring tendons are located in the back of the knee.

In either instance, you address it the same way. I'm always a fan of starting with self-massage techniques on page 83 to create immediate change. From there, you can try the sciatic nerve glides (more on the sciatic nerve and sciatica on page 67) and gentle hamstring stretching to increase flexibility.

From there, you can move on to the hamstring exercises listed at the end of this section. If you are able to stay consistent and avoid long periods of sitting, everything should improve quickly.

CALF TENDINITIS/TENDINOSIS

In your calf, you have two main muscle groups: the gastrocnemius and the soleus. The gastrocnemius is the muscle with tendons that cross the back of the knee and can therefore be responsible for pain in that area.

It is far more common for tightness in the calf to cause pain either directly over the muscle or down at its lower attachment, the Achilles tendon. In either instance, any pain caused by the calf is dealt with in the same way.

You can find out what to do by reading "The Calf" section (see page 36) along with the "Achilles Tendinitis/Tendinosis" section (see page 29).

BAKER'S CYST

If tightness in the gastrocnemius and soleus muscle groups is present for long enough, you can start to develop something known as a Baker's cyst. This is a small nodule that can develop right in the back of the knee and will often be extremely sensitive to the touch and cause significant discomfort when fully bending the knee. You will often be able to feel this nodule, and the more irritated it gets, the larger it will be.

In most cases, the cyst can be reduced and symptoms can be cleared by following all of the same techniques listed for hamstring and calf tightness starting on page 85. If you focus on increasing the strength and flexibility of the calf and hamstring for four to six weeks and the cyst is still present and painful, it would be a good idea to seek advice from a sports medicine MD to see if more measures need to be taken to shrink the cyst.

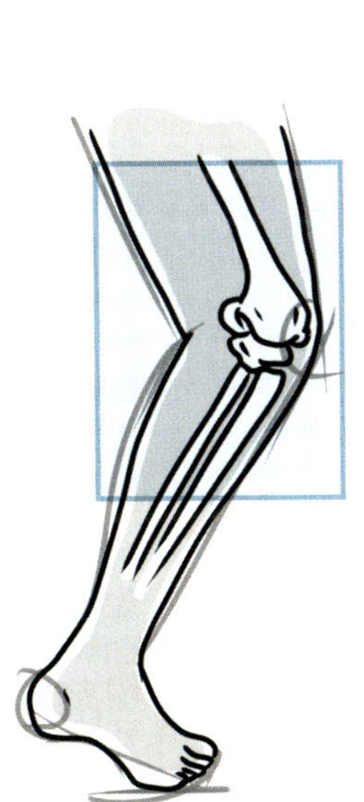

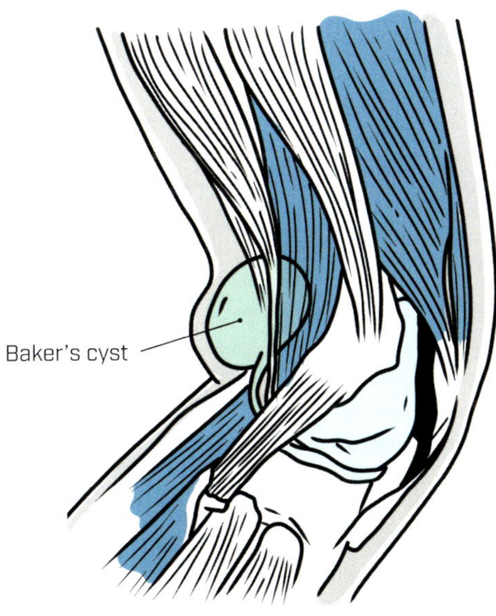

THE THIGH

As discussed elsewhere in this book, a muscle is most likely to cause pain where the tendons attach to bone. While feeling tightness in the muscle itself is common, the actual pain is often at the ends of muscles close to the joints that they cross. Because of this, you can find out what to do about tightness in the thigh muscles by referring to the sections that correspond to the areas that are most likely to be causing pain:

- **For tightness in the quads,** see the section on pain in the front of the knee (page 50).
- **For tightness along the outside of the leg,** see the section on IT band pain (page 63).
- **For tightness along the inside of the leg,** see the sections on pes anserine pain (page 60) and groin pain (page 74).
- **For tightness along the back of the thigh,** read through the previous entry on the hamstring and calf (page 64).

SCIATICA

Sciatica is an increasingly common diagnosis that, when present, can be debilitating. It is known for causing burning, tingling, or tightness along the back of the leg.

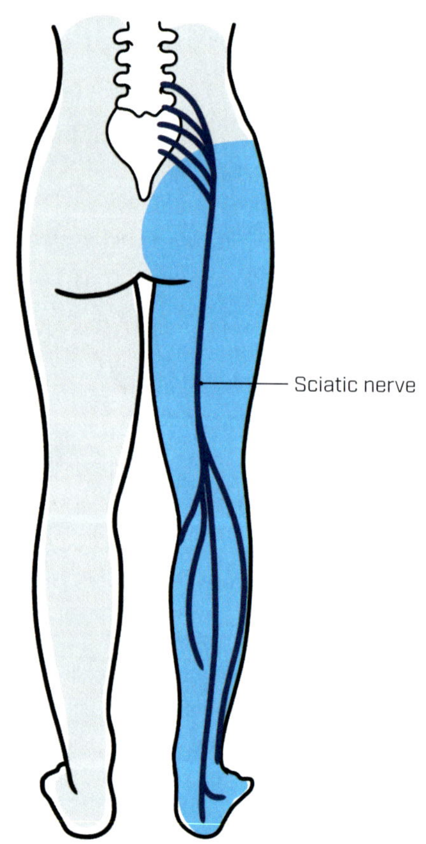

The sciatic nerve is the biggest nerve in your body. Made up of the nerve roots that leave lumbar levels 4 and 5 and sacral levels 1-3, it travels down the back of the leg until it gets to the knee, where it splits off into smaller branches. The two most common sources of what is called sciatica or sciatic pain are the lower back itself (which you can read about in the lower back section) and piriformis syndrome (which you can read about in the hip section). Both sources cause irritation in the nerve, and you may end up feeling a burning, tingling, or painful sensation anywhere from the upper butt area all the way down to the calf.

To improve symptoms, there is one exercise that works for almost all cases. It's called the sciatic nerve glide, and you can read exactly how to do it on page 000.

The key to this nerve-gliding exercise is to be very gentle and not spend too long at the point of tension. Sciatic nerve pain can feel a lot like hamstring tightness to some people, but if you try to stretch it out, you will only increase the symptoms. Nerves follow a very different set of rules than muscles, and if you try to outstretch a nerve issue, the nerve will always win.

The sciatic nerve gets a lot of shine because of how many different nerve roots comprise it, but all of the nerves that leave the lower back can cause discomfort somewhere in the legs. And since those nerves innervate very specific places, where you feel the pain can point you directly to where the issue lies.

This dermatome map shows which nerves supply feeling to which areas in the leg. As mentioned earlier, the sciatic nerve comprises nerve endings from L4 through S3, but there are more nerves that supply sensation to the legs. And if you have a consistent burning, tingling, or painful sensation in a very particular part of your leg, this map can point you to the exact nerve that is wreaking havoc. For most of these specific pains, the true root of the problem is where the nerve starts in the lower back, which you can read more about in the lower back section on page 94.

Lower Body Dermatome Map

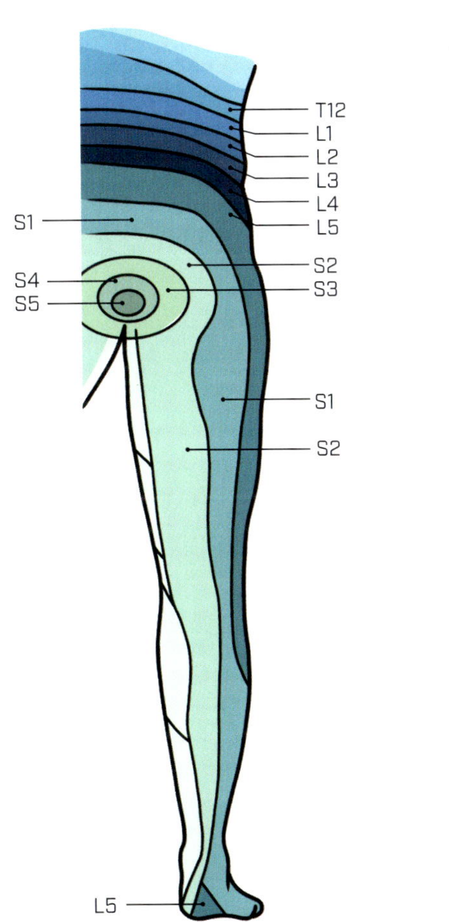

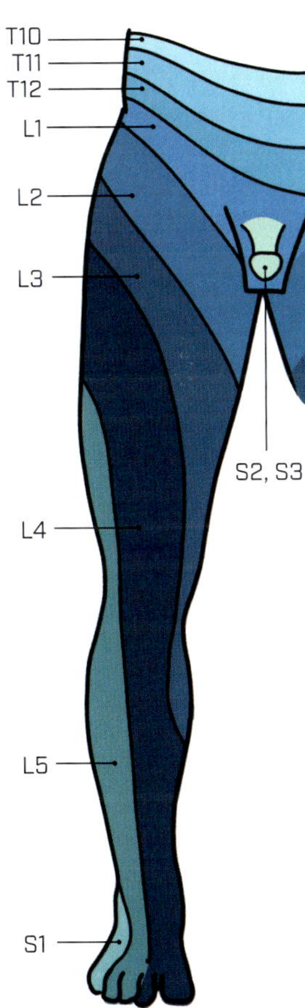

The 4 Muscular Zones

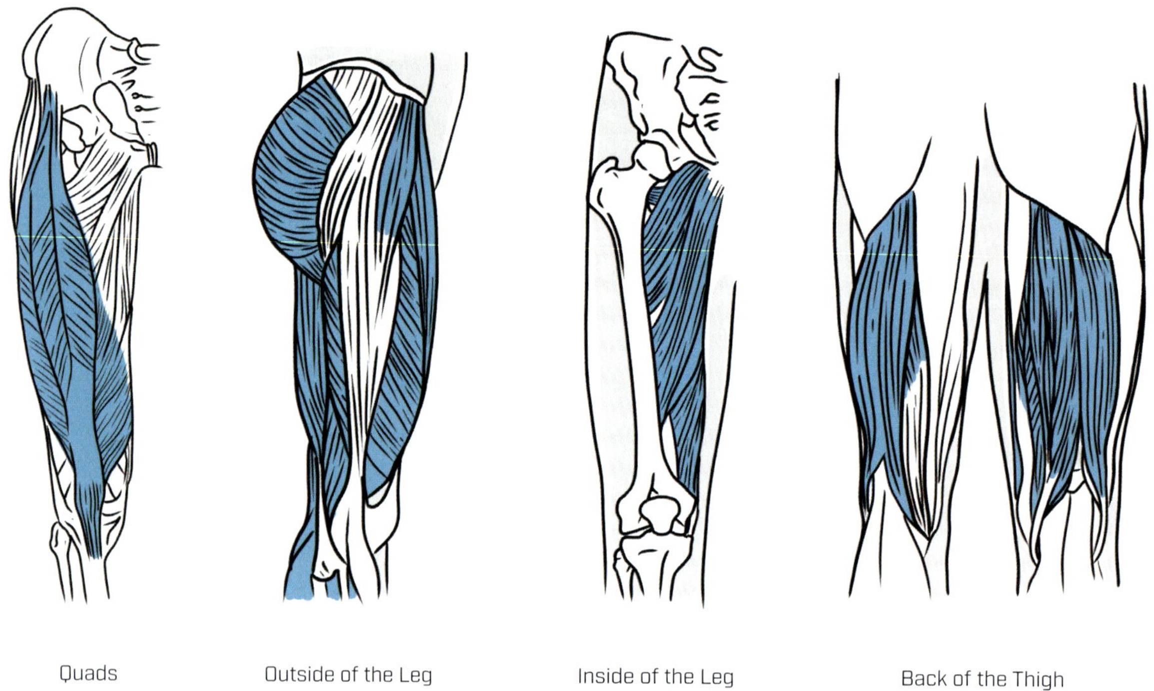

Quads Outside of the Leg Inside of the Leg Back of the Thigh

THE HIP

The hip is the largest joint in the body and arguably the most important. Not only can the hip itself be in pain, but when there is pain in the lower back or knee, building strength and mobility in the hip is the best way to regain control over those two areas. That's a lot of responsibility for one joint! It lies right near the middle of your center of gravity, and because of the massive muscles that control it, the hip can truly be thought of as the command center for the lower half of the body.

It can be broken up into four main zones. The hip flexors are in the front, the hip abductors are on the outside, the hip adductors are on the inside, and the hip extensors make up the back side. Any one of these four muscular zones can be solely responsible for your discomfort, and you can read more about them in their individual sections.

Other than the muscular component, since the hip is a "ball and socket" joint, it also has a labrum. The labrum can be thought of as a suction cup made of fibrocartilage that wraps around the head of the femur where it fits into the pelvis. And because an issue with the labrum of the hip can cause discomfort throughout the hip, that is where we will start.

Hip Labral Tear

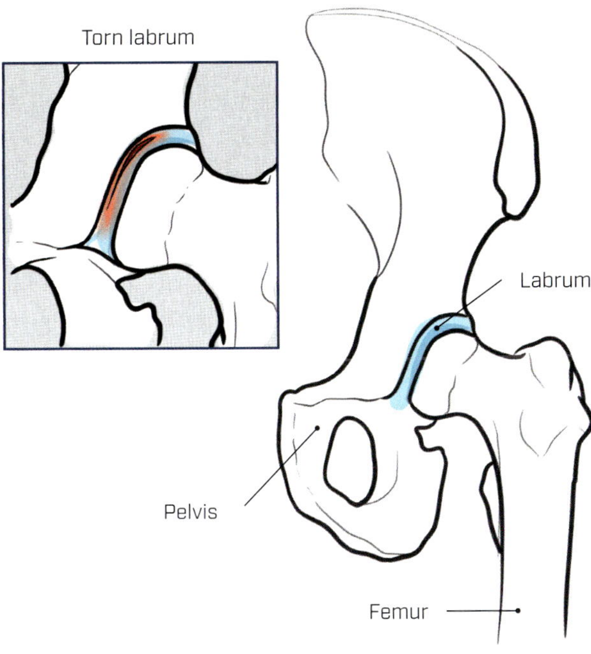

LABRUM TEAR

The labrum is the main source of structural stability in the hip, so if it is compromised, it becomes much more important to build the strength and stability of the musculature. A tear in the labrum of the hip can occur in one of two main ways. The first way is less common and results from a traumatic injury. An event where you plant and twist your leg while your leg is stuck to the ground, like a football player trying to evade a defender, could cause a tear. A car accident where there is a quick and powerful force directed at the hip or leg might also cause one.

The more common way to injure the labrum of the hip is to do it slowly over time. It is more common in flexible people who frequently test the end ranges of their hips, like dancers, but can also develop in anyone who has spent the bulk of their life being active and athletic.

No matter how you hurt it, the symptoms will largely present in the same way. When there is a tear in the labrum, it is common to feel a frequent popping or clicking when moving the hip, and the hip may feel like it gets "stuck." It is also common for the hip to feel unstable and sometimes buckle while also creating a pinching pain and discomfort when trying to bring your knee to your chest or across your body. You may feel pain in some specific places "deep" in the hip, but it is also common to feel a "C-shaped" pain, or a pain that wraps around the outside of the hip and is felt deep inside.

C-Shaped Pain

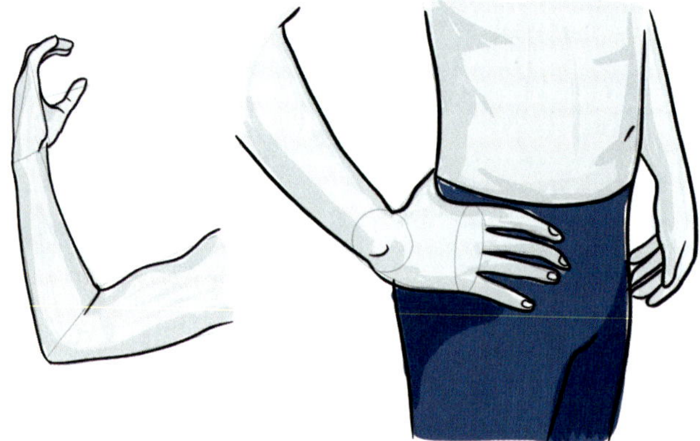

If your pain is severe and limiting and you have never gotten an official diagnosis, it may be a good idea to see an orthopedic or sports medicine MD to assess the severity of the tear. But if you already know you have a tear, or if the pain is manageable, the best first step is to try to build strength and control.

It is best to work the muscles in all four zones, avoiding the exercises that involve rotation at the beginning. Start with hip flexion, abduction, and extension exercises, making sure that you aren't increasing your pain or feeling painful popping or clicking. Keep the range of motion of the exercises small enough that you feel like you are fatiguing the muscles but not increasing any of your symptoms.

If working on that for a few weeks starts to make a big difference, you can then progress to more challenging compound movements like squats and lunges and start to add in some exercises that work the hip rotators. Once again, it is important to start small and build up slowly over time, and, as always, if no progress is being made, you should see a professional in person.

FEMORAL ACETABULAR IMPINGEMENT (FAI) / HIP IMPINGEMENT

Another common cause of "C-shaped" pain is an impingement created by either the femur or the acetabulum in the front of the hip. The head of the femur sits in the acetabulum, which is located on your pelvis, and the two of them make up the "ball and socket" portions of the hip joint, the acetabulum being the socket and the head of the femur being the ball. When you have an impingement, you will likely experience discomfort when trying to bring your knee to your chest or across your body. You may feel discomfort when trying to get into a deep squat as well. It is also common for impingements to be associated with labral tears.

The two deformities that can lead to an FAI are a cam deformity (a growth on the femur) and a pincer deformity (a growth on the acetabulum). You can't know for sure which one you have without an X-ray, and technically the only way to take away these deformities is with surgery.

Cam and Pincer Deformities

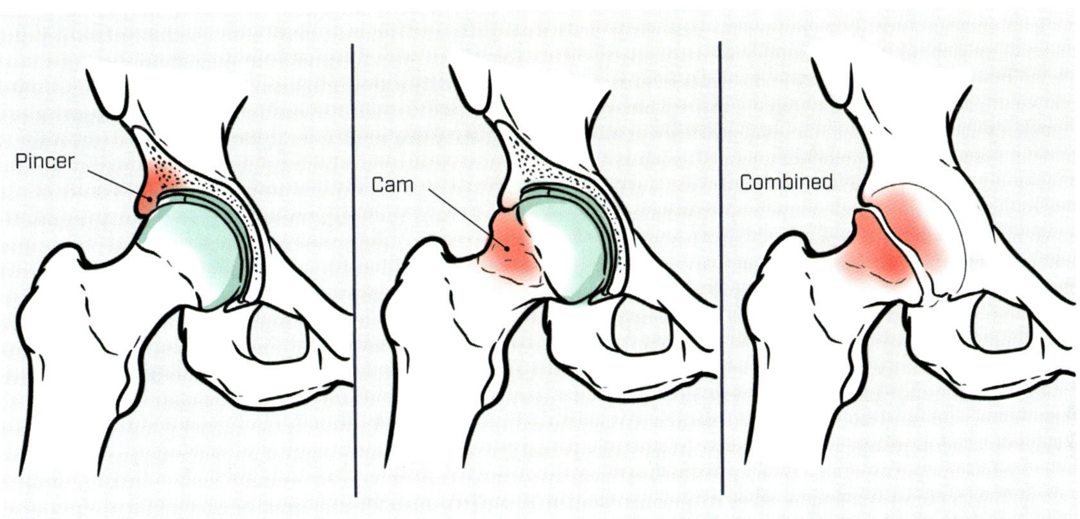

But if you learn nothing else from this book, I hope you at least learn that no matter what is seen on imaging, and no matter what can or can't be changed anatomically, you can almost always improve your symptoms, strength, and function. In the case of FAI, while some of your symptoms may be coming from the impingement, in my experience, most of the symptoms come from tightness and weakness in the surrounding musculature. And by using the self-massage techniques along with the strengthening techniques found at the end of this section, you can make a massive improvement in how your hip feels on a regular basis.

Just make sure that when going through the exercises, you are feeling muscle fatigue but no increase in symptoms. Stay consistent and build up slowly; always listen to your body, and don't fight into pain. And since this is so closely associated with labral tears (see page 69), be sure to read that section as well.

THE FRONT OF THE HIP

The hip flexors are a group of three muscles that cross the front of the hip. If you're feeling pain or discomfort in the front of the hip that doesn't align with the previously mentioned labral tear or hip impingement, then you may have an issue with your hip flexors.

HIP FLEXOR PAIN AND TIGHTNESS

The hip flexor muscle group is made up of the psoas, iliacus, and rectus femoris. Since they work as a unit for the most part, if you're having trouble with one, you're having trouble with all of them.

Hip Flexor Muscle Group

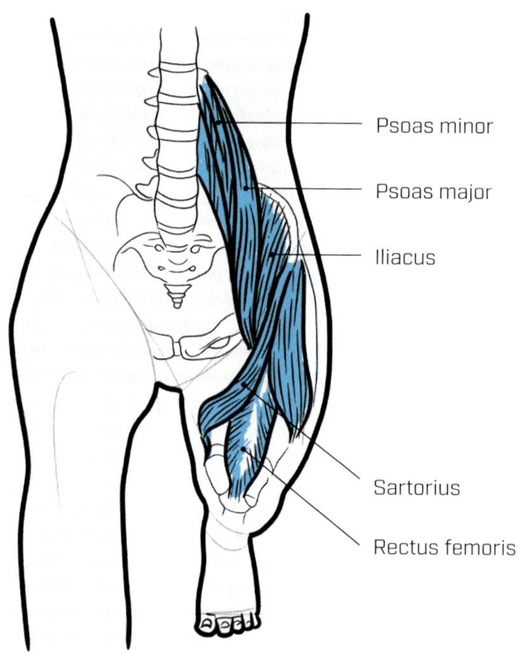

Issues with the hip flexor have become very common because tightness and weakness can develop with prolonged sitting. When sitting, your hip flexors are in a shortened position, and since most of us sit while working and sit in our free time after work, it's not hard to imagine why so many people experience tightness in their hip flexors.

There is a muscle that is not a true hip flexor muscle but lies just to the side of the hip flexors, called the tensor fascia latae (TFL). It's the pesky and stubborn muscle that is the main attachment of the IT band. If you're feeling pain in this muscle and it hasn't responded to the hip flexor stretches and exercises, please read the "Iliotibial (IT) Band Pain" section (see page 63) to make sure you are also addressing the TFL.

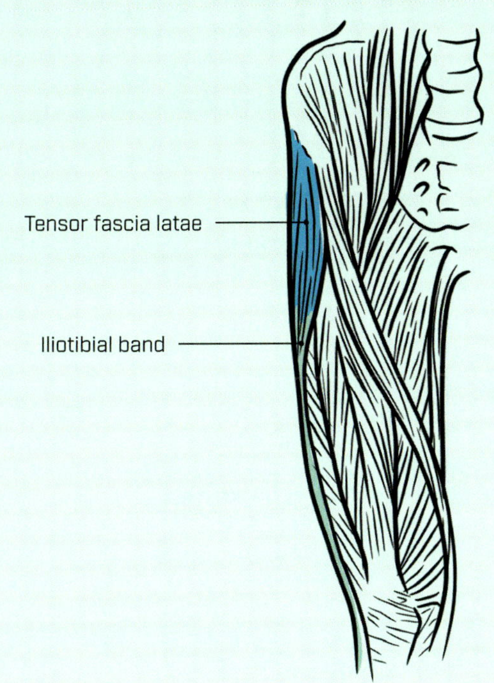

If you feel a tightness across the front of the hip, especially when standing up after having been sitting for a while, it's probably caused by tightness and weakness in your hip flexor. You may also feel an increase in tightness and discomfort after walking for a prolonged period of time. If this muscle group becomes irritated enough, you may even feel pressure when trying to bring your knee to your chest or feel a deep "snapping" sensation in the hip when raising your leg.

If you suspect that your hip flexors are an issue, the first thing to do is to try to spend less time sitting. The more you get up throughout the day, the better. While you're taking more standing breaks, you can also mix in the hip flexor stretch found at the end of this section on page 87. If you do even one set of this stretch every time you stand up, you should start to feel a big difference fairly quickly.

Other than stretching, it's also important that you strengthen the hip flexors. There are a few options at the end of the section, and it would be a good idea to work on these movements two to three days a week.

Finally, tightness in the hip flexor can be exacerbated if you are lacking hip internal rotation. So, mix in some of the hip internal rotation exercises two to three times a week.

THE INSIDE OF THE HIP (GROIN AREA)

The inside of the hip is an extremely sensitive area where pain can be incredibly uncomfortable. It is primarily the adductor group that causes muscular issues, but there are some other issues to look out for. Before reading this section, please review the rundown on labrum tears and hip impingements at the start of the hip section, as those issues are common causes of discomfort deep on the inside of the hip. If you feel like what you're dealing with is more in the groin area, then let's dive right in.

GROIN/ADDUCTOR STRAIN OR TIGHTNESS

The muscles that make up the groin area are known as the adductors, and they are a group of five muscles that more or less work in tandem. The longest adductor muscle runs all the way down past the knee, and the shortest doesn't travel very far at all.

The 5 Adductor Muscles

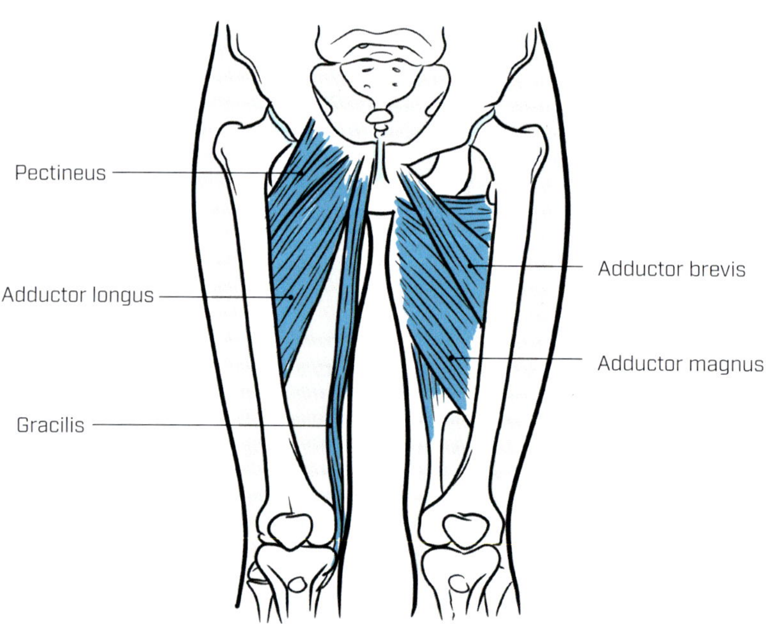

In my experience, this muscle group becomes injured in two main ways. The first is a traumatic injury, where you may have quickly lunged to the side or tried to pull your leg in while your foot was planted on the ground. In that case, you may feel immediate pain in the groin muscles that will persist for a few weeks. The best way to start to address this discomfort is with very gentle adductor stretches and some easy adductor exercises that you can find on page 86. It is important to start gently and make sure that the stretches and exercises aren't increasing your symptoms. Once your flexibility and strength begin to return, you can progress to more challenging exercises.

The second main cause of adductor pain happens slowly over time. It can occur due to a lack of mobility or strength in other areas of the hip, so the groin ends up taking on too much work. You may feel this pain when running, jogging, or walking or at the bottom of a lunge or deep squat. While it is still a good idea to do the adductor stretches and exercises, in order to address the root cause of this pain, it is also important to improve your hip internal rotation and the strength of your hip abductors. These movements can be found at the end of this section. As you improve strength and mobility, it is important to make sure that you have the ability to use other muscle groups when going through those more challenging movements. Over time, the adductor muscles should calm down, and you should feel more even throughout your hip.

INGUINAL HERNIA

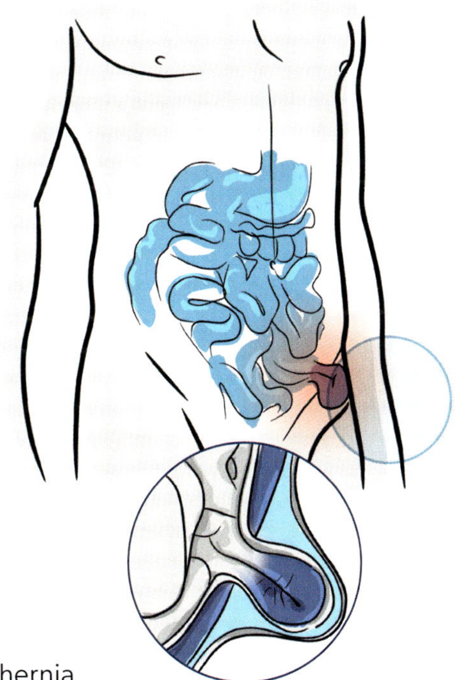

If you're experiencing pain high up in the groin area that started after you tried to lift a heavy object or strained to do a tough task, it is important to rule out an inguinal hernia. An inguinal hernia develops when something in your abdomen, like an intestine, breaks through a weak spot in your inguinal canal and protrudes through the body.

In the case of a large hernia, you will be able to see and feel the spot where it took place. In the case of a smaller hernia, or if you have a lot of fatty tissue in that area, it may take a CT scan to diagnose. But if the pain started while straining and you continue to feel pain when straining, lifting, or even coughing or sneezing, it is a good idea to make an appointment with your MD.

While people sometimes feel comfortable living with a small hernia, the only way to truly fix the issue is with surgery to rebuild the part of the abdominal wall where the hernia took place.

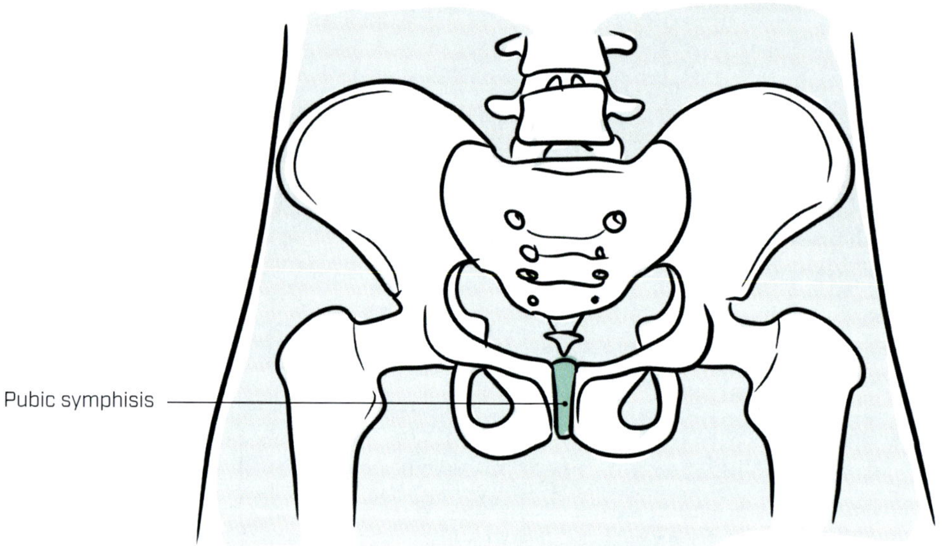

PUBIC PAIN

If your pain is more toward the middle of your pelvis, then the issue may be your pubic symphysis. This is rare, but if you are hypermobile, or especially if you have given birth, there may be enough movement happening in this area to create pain. You can use the illustration to help find the pubic symphysis on yourself, and if you're able to replicate your pain simply by pushing over that spot, there's a good chance that is what you're dealing with.

If this area is in pain, it is likely because it is moving too much. In order to reduce that pain, you have to reintroduce stability in the muscles in this area. The best exercises for this purpose are the three Pilates ring exercises found at the end of the lower back section on page 106. Once you can comfortably complete those exercises, you can then progress to the hip exercises found at the end of this section. As long as you progress slowly, the stability from the muscles should hopefully greatly reduce the pain in the pubic area.

Hip Abductors

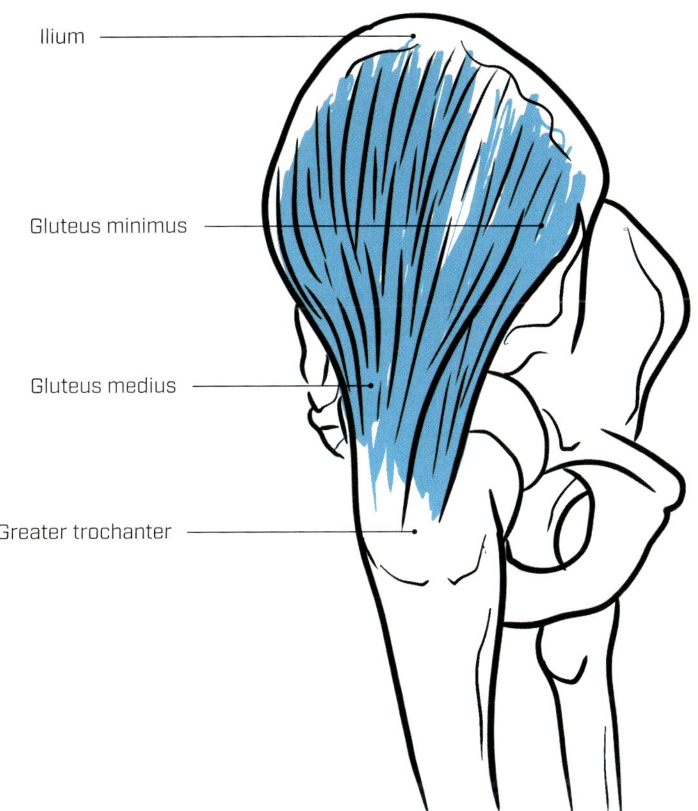

THE OUTSIDE OF THE HIP

Working on building strength in the outside of the hip is discussed at length throughout this book. Not only are the hip abductors extremely important to reducing knee pain, but, since they are your primary pelvic stabilizers, they are influential in pelvic and lower back pain as well. So, if you've already browsed through the sections on the knee and lower back, you are probably well acquainted with the muscles discussed in this section.

While the muscles on the outside of the hip can cause problems both up and down the chain of the body, this section is reserved for what it feels like when they are causing a problem right at home.

GREATER TROCHANTER BURSITIS

The greater trochanter (GT) is the epicenter of all the muscles that lie on the outside of the hip. It is a bony prominence on the side of your femur where a lot of these muscles share an attachment point. When the GT is inflamed, it will get to the point where you can no longer put any pressure on that area, making lying on your side an extremely unpleasant experience. You can use the illustration to find the GT on yourself, and if pressing over that bony prominence recreates your pain, then that's likely what you're dealing with.

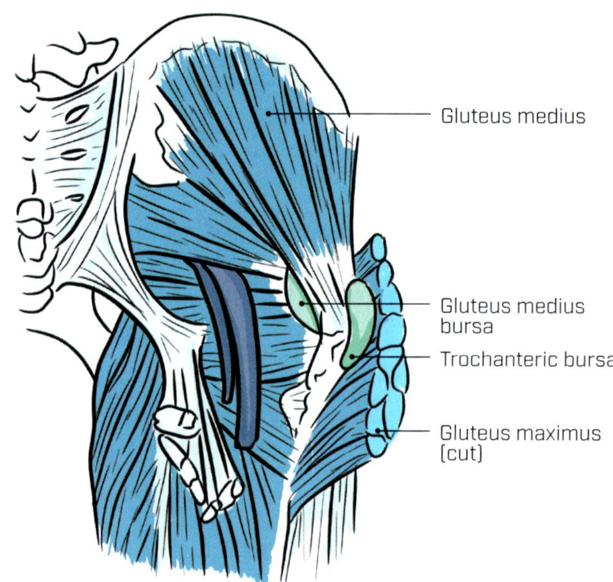

If you don't have pain directly over the GT but you do have pain and tenderness in the muscles that attach to the GT, then following the advice in this section is still a good idea. Pain over the GT may only develop when tightness in the musculature has been around for a long time. Following the advice found here can hopefully reduce pain in the surrounding muscles and stop the pain over the GT from developing in the first place.

The best place to start to reduce symptoms is with the self-massage techniques for these muscles that you can find on page 83. It's best to stick with the handheld roller or the massage gun, making sure that you're using firm yet gentle pressure and staying on the muscles and off the GT itself. In fact, it is best to avoid any sort of pressure over the GT to allow the inflammation to go down.

Once pain and discomfort start to diminish, you can begin to do the strengthening exercises. Start small and build up slowly, but as you improve the strength of these muscles, the wear and tear taking place at the GT should greatly reduce.

ILIOTIBIAL [IT] BAND PAIN [HIP]

While the most common presentation of IT band pain is either at the bottom of the IT band on the outside of the knee or along the outside of the thigh, sometimes the IT band causes pain on the outside of the hip, where it crosses paths with the GT. If you feel a clicking sensation right over the GT while doing something like climbing stairs or pedaling a bike, then this is the more likely source. Since the IT band crosses over the GT, if there is tension in the system, it can cause a click every time the hip goes through a certain range of motion.

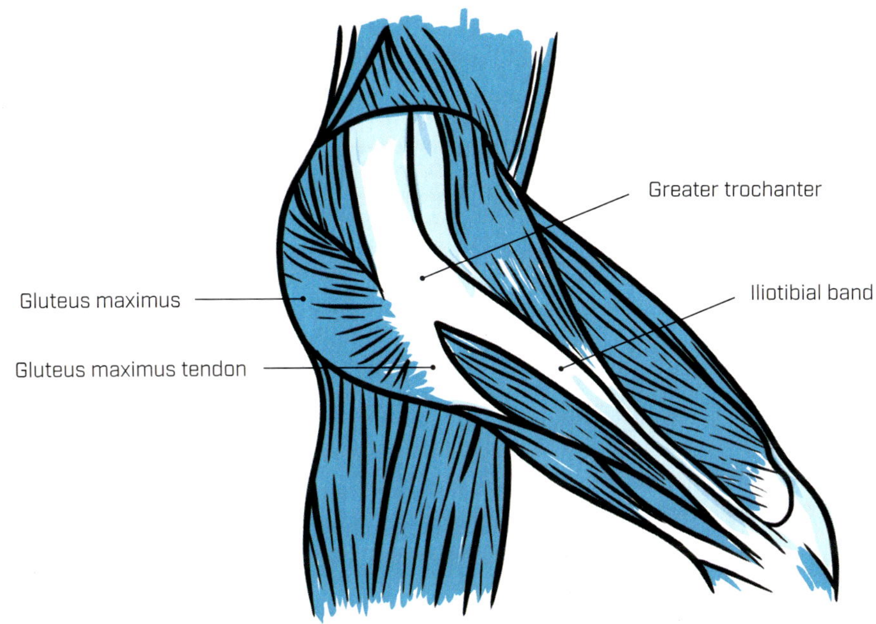

For more information on the IT band and what you can do to reduce symptoms, please refer to the section "The Outside of the Knee" (see page 62).

THE BACK OF THE HIP

The back side of the hip gets a lot of publicity. If you're an Instagram model, it may be your main source of attention. If you're an athlete, it's your main source of power. If you're a child, it's your main source of humor.

No matter what the backside means to you, you should think of it as a very important part of your body. Your glutes are the biggest and most powerful muscles that you have, and when used correctly, they not only make you more athletic, functional, and capable but can also greatly reduce pain throughout your body. That is precisely why so many diagnoses discussed in this book come with a recommendation to improve glute strength.

Since this muscle group is so influential, I would go so far as to say that if you could work on only one muscle group to reduce pain anywhere from the lower back down, it would be the glutes. But when you're feeling pain directly in the backside itself, here's what you can do.

HAMSTRING TENDINITIS TENDINOSIS/TIGHTNESS

While it is more common for the hamstring to create pain down at its lower attachment site behind the knee or over the muscle belly itself, sometimes it can create pain at its upper attachment in the back side of the hip. That attachment site is called your ischial tuberosity and is the bony part of your butt that you sit on.

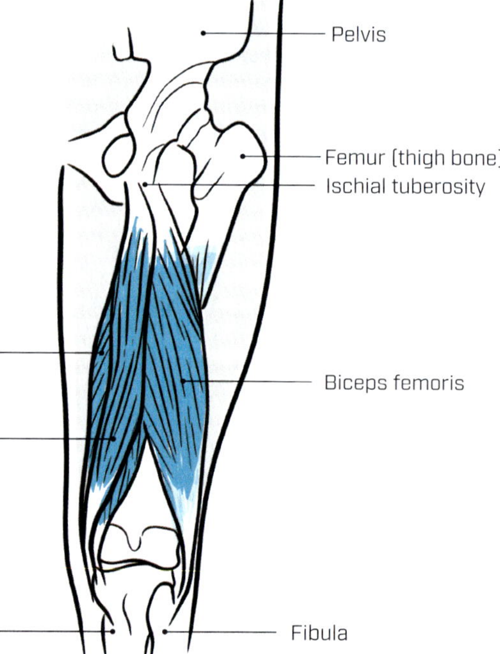

Since the hamstring is the biggest and most influential thing that attaches to this bony area, if you are experiencing pain there, it's the most likely cause. To learn more about what to do for the hamstring, you can go back to where it is discussed in the section "The Back of the Knee" (see page 63).

But when you are feeling pain in this area, it is also important to work on the glute exercises at the end of this section. And when doing these exercises, it's important to try to squeeze and use the glute as much as you can while trying to avoid that work coming from the hamstring. Learning how to use the glutes without feeling like you're overworking the hamstring takes a lot of stress and strain off the hamstrings. If you're able to integrate the advice from this section and the knee section, you should hopefully experience a significant reduction in pain.

PIRIFORMIS PAIN

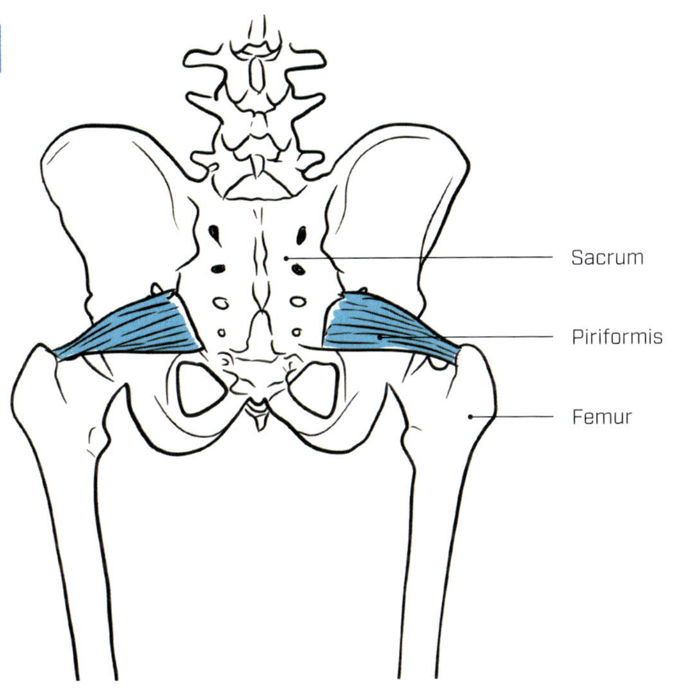

If the pain that you're feeling is a little higher up and feels like more of a muscular tightness, then you may be having pain in your piriformis. The piriformis is a muscle that runs horizontally across the backside, and due to its proximity to the sciatic nerve, it can be quite the troublemaker. When it is tight, you may feel the discomfort right where it is in the glute area or at its attachment points in the GT or the sacrum.

When experiencing piriformis pain, the best first step is to start doing the piriformis stretches found at the end of this section. Keep the stretches gentle, and make sure that when finishing a stretch, you feel an improvement in symptoms. If you find that symptoms increase, it means that you are pushing them too far.

As the stretches start to improve symptoms, it is also important to do exercises for the glutes and the hip abductors to help take strain away from the piriformis. And since the piriformis does lie so close to the sciatic nerve, it is also a good idea to read the section on sciatica and follow the advice listed there (see page 67).

SACROILIAC (SI) JOINT PAIN

The SI joint is right in the middle of your two gluteal areas, and most people probably think of it as the lower back. But since it is at the same level as the glutes, I am including it here. In most people, the SI joint will not be an issue, because in most people, the SI joint is fully fused. However, if you are hypermobile, a dancer who does frequent kicks and splits, or someone who has given birth, then the SI joint may be mobile enough to create pain.

When experiencing pain in the SI joint, people will most likely feel it along the edges of the sacrum, and pain will be increased when doing things like bending over at the waist or twisting.

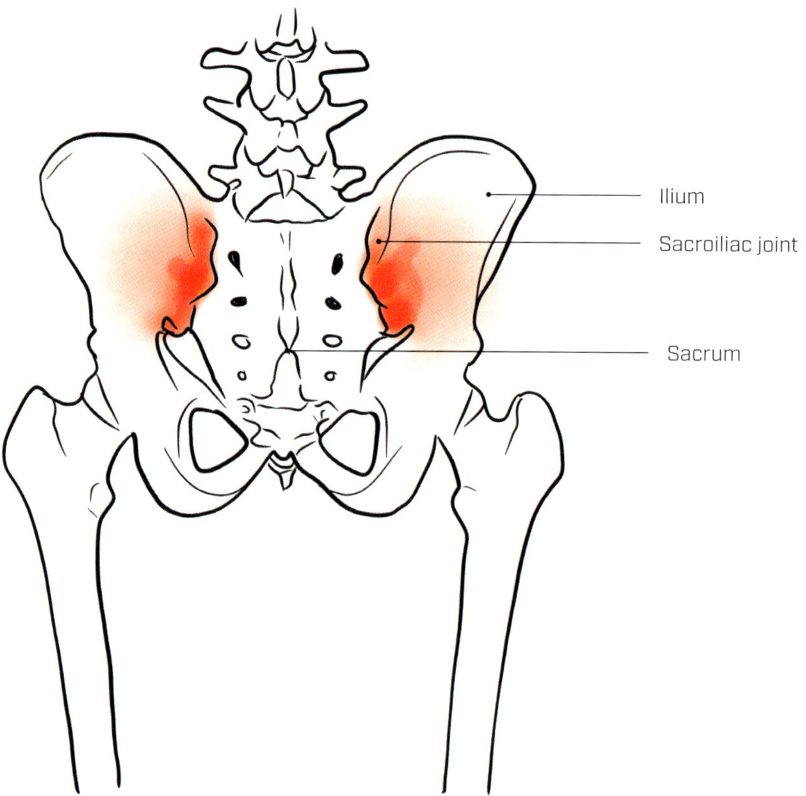

Since the pain that comes from the SI joint is mostly due to excess movement, the best way to start to reduce pain is by introducing stability. The best way to do so is to perform the three Pilates ring movements found at the end of the lower back section (see page 106). As your symptoms begin to ease, you can start to work on the other hip exercises found at the end of this section. Just make sure to start small and build up slowly.

SCIATIC NERVE / GENERAL NERVE PAIN

If what you're feeling in the back of your hip is more of a numbness, tingling, or burning, then what you are feeling is likely nerve related. To learn more about this pain, make sure to read the section on sciatica on page 67 and the section on the lower back starting on page 95 to learn how an issue there can lead to nerve pain felt farther down the chain.

SELF-MASSAGE TECHNIQUES & MOBILITY, FLEXIBILITY, AND STRENGTHENING MOVEMENTS FOR THE KNEE, THIGH, AND HIP

SELF-MASSAGE

HANDHELD ROLLER

A handheld roller is best used for the larger muscle groups in this region, such as the quads, adductors, and hamstrings. This is easiest to do while sitting in a chair, making sure that the muscle group you're working on is completely relaxed. Spend three to five minutes on whatever muscle group you're targeting, focusing on tight areas you find along the way. Use firm but gentle pressure, and make sure that when you're done, you feel better than when you started. If you feel sore or bruised afterward, you were pressing too hard.

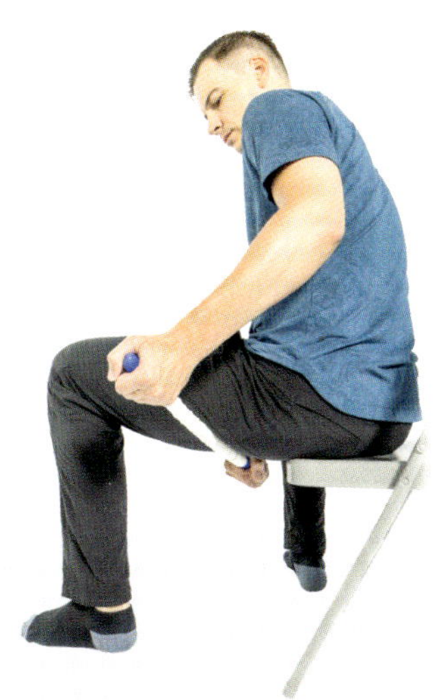

MASSAGE GUN

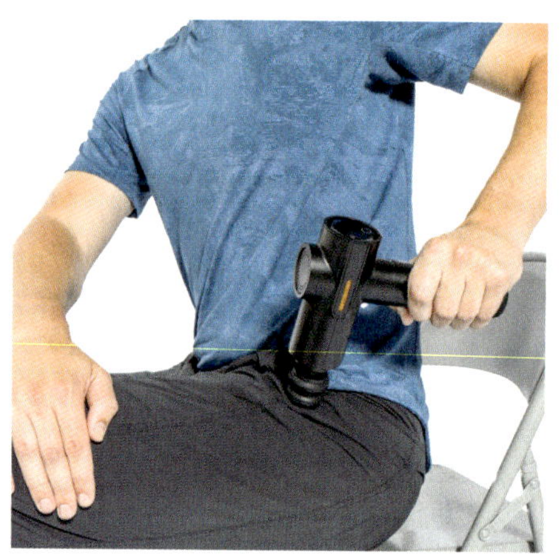

For the smaller muscles like the TFL and the muscles along the side of the hip, it is easier to use a massage gun. You can do it sitting in a chair, making sure that the muscles you're working on are relaxed. Spend two to four minutes on the muscle you are targeting, applying a firm downward pressure with the massage gun. Be sure to stay over muscles and never go over bony areas. Start with a gentle setting to make sure it isn't too much for the muscle. If you ever feel sore or bruised after using a massage gun, you were either pressing too hard or using a setting that was too high.

MOBILITY

HIP INTERNAL ROTATION

Lying on your back, keep your knees bent with your feet spread apart. Keep your lower back glued to the floor while lowering the inside of one knee down toward the floor until you feel a slight stretch. Once you feel a slight stretch, bring it back out and repeat with the other leg. Do roughly ten to fifteen repetitions.

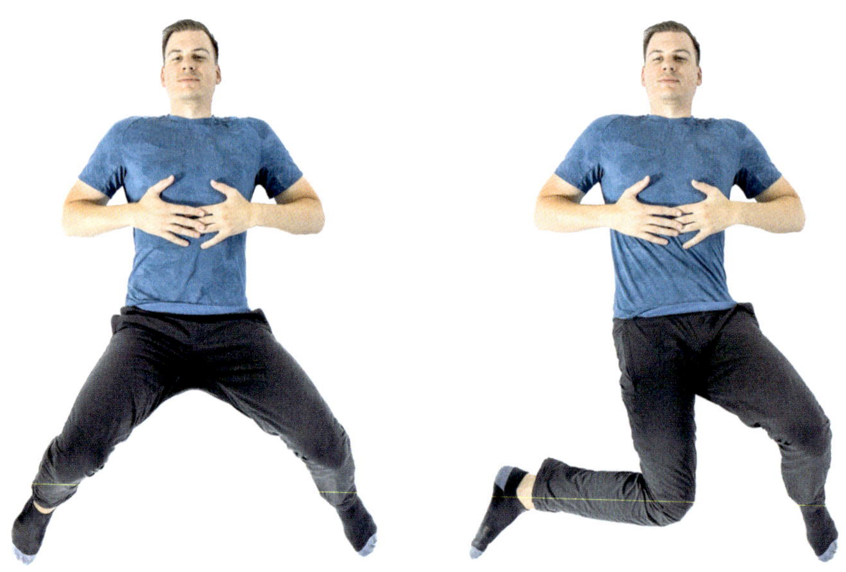

SCIATIC NERVE GLIDES

Lying on your back, grasp behind one of your legs with both hands. Keeping your toes pointed toward your face, slowly straighten your knee until you feel a slight stretch in the back of your leg. Only go until you feel a gentle stretch, and don't worry about trying to fully straighten your knee. Hold for a second before returning to the starting position. Do two sets of fifteen on each leg.

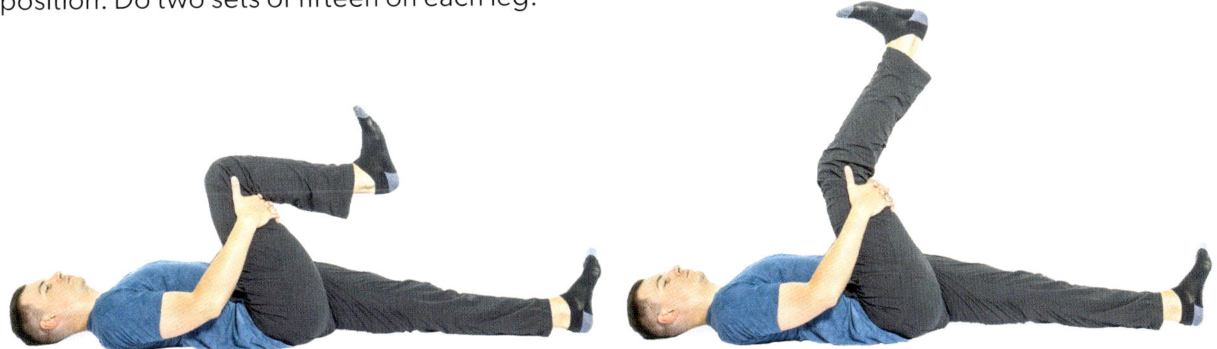

FLEXIBILITY

HAMSTRING STRETCH

Sit up tall on the edge of a chair and extend one leg out in front of you. Keep your heel on the ground with the front of your foot raised and a slight bend in the knee. With your chest tall and lower back extended, simply bend over at the waist until you feel a gentle stretch in your hamstring. Hold for fifteen to twenty seconds and repeat three times.

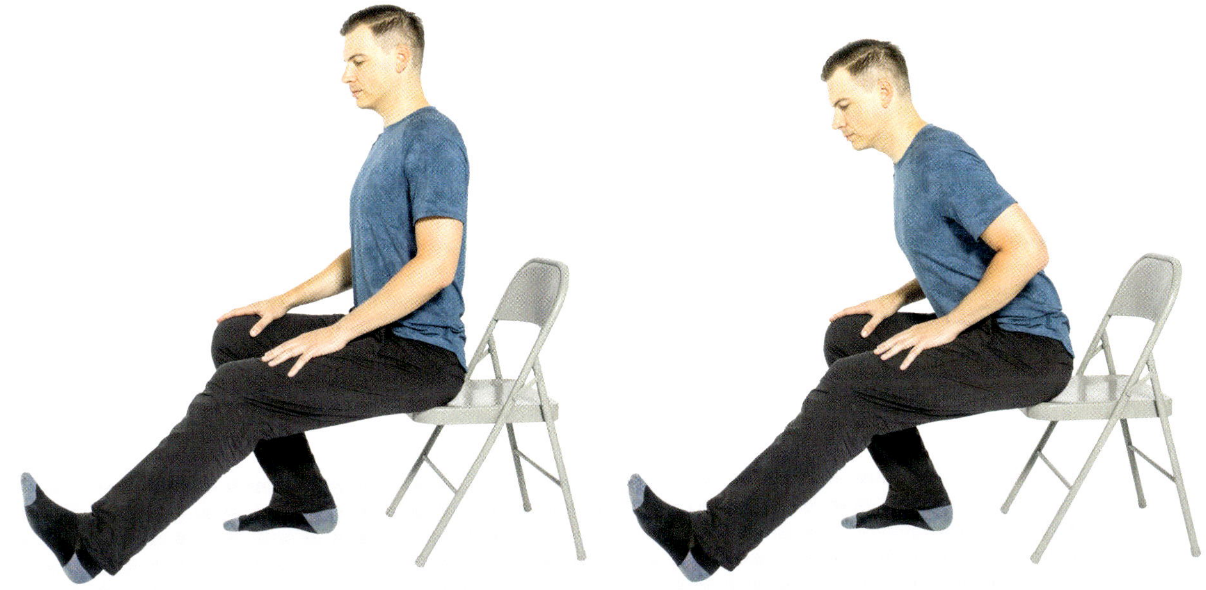

QUAD STRETCH

Standing up and holding onto something for support, grab your foot behind you with the opposite hand. Stand tall until you feel a gentle stretch in the front of your leg. Once you feel a gentle stretch, hold for fifteen to twenty seconds and repeat three times.

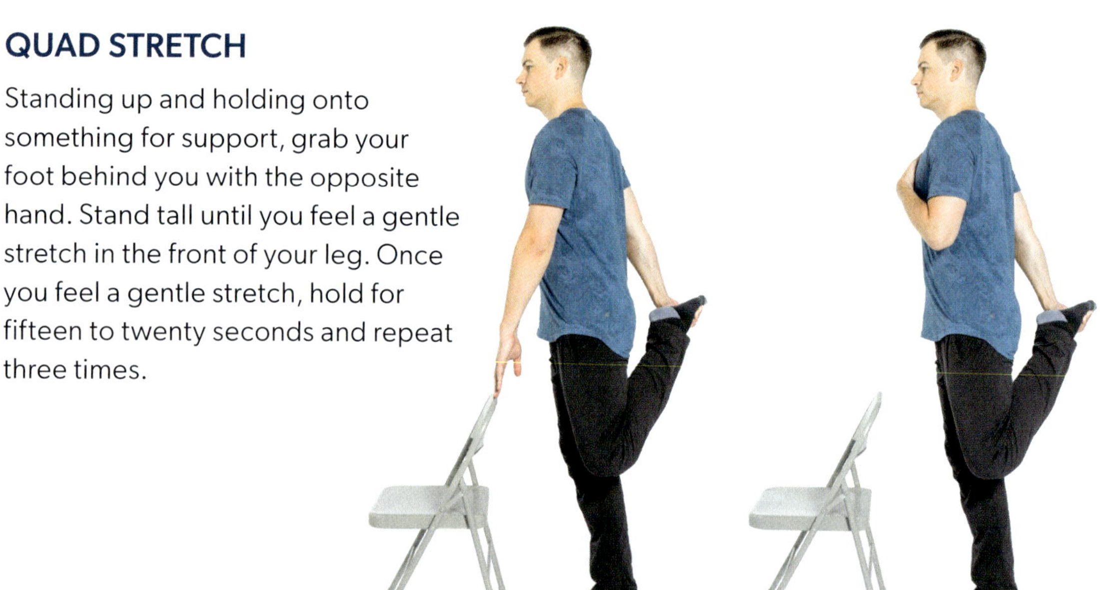

HIP ADDUCTOR STRETCH

Stand with your feet slightly wider than shoulder-width apart. Keep your feet grounded on the floor as you tilt your pelvis toward the side you want to stretch. You should be able to feel a stretch just by tilting your pelvis, but if you want to increase the stretch, you can lunge slightly to the opposite side. Once you feel a gentle stretch, hold for fifteen to twenty seconds and repeat three times.

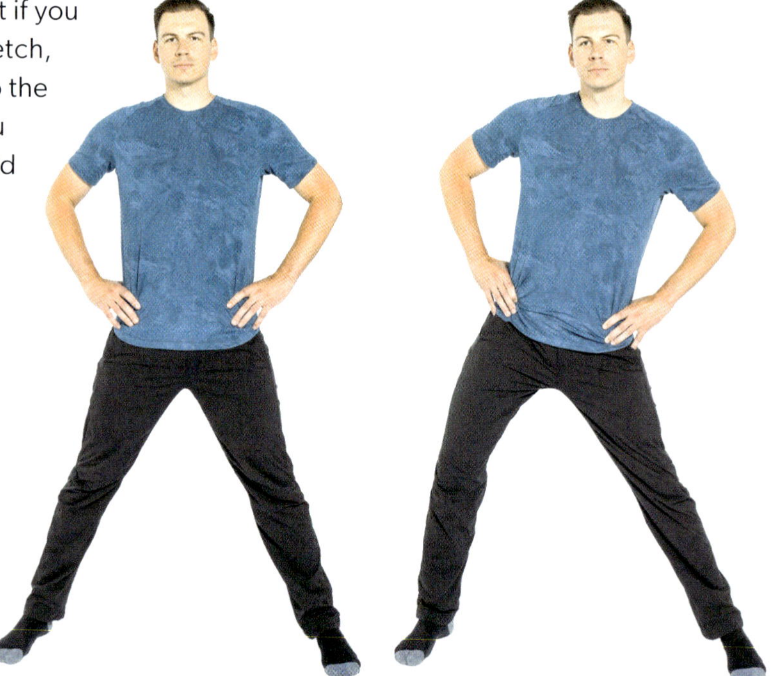

HIP FLEXOR STRETCH

Stand in a staggered stance with the leg you want to stretch in back. Push the front of the hip of the back leg forward while squeezing your glute on that side. You should feel a stretch in the front of the hip with just that action, but to increase the stretch, you can raise the arm of the side you are stretching up over your head. Once you feel a gentle stretch, hold for fifteen to twenty seconds and repeat three times.

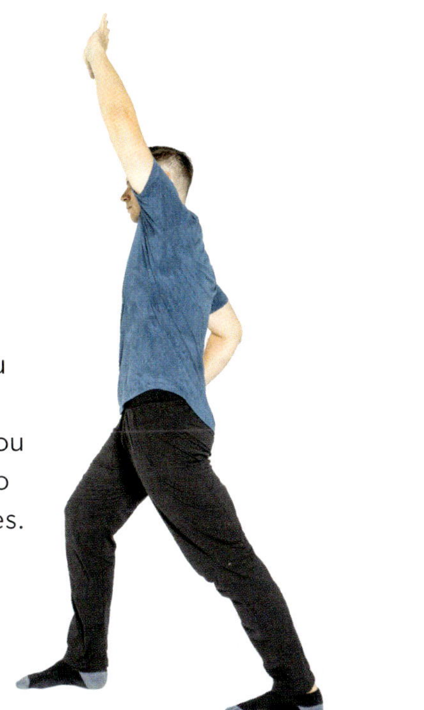

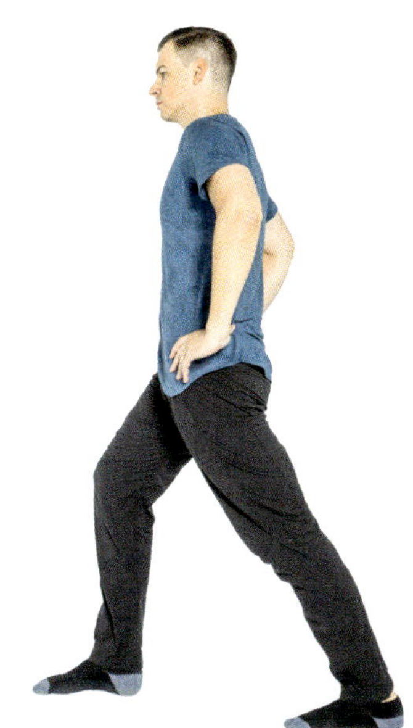

PIRIFORMIS STRETCH

Lying on your back with both knees bent, place the ankle of the leg you want to stretch on your opposite knee. Grab onto the knee of the leg you want to stretch and pull it up and across your body toward your opposite shoulder until you feel a stretch in the back of your hip. If you don't feel a stretch in the back of the hip and only feel pressure in the front of the hip, instead of pulling your leg across your body, just take one hand and push that leg forward until you feel a stretch in the back of the hip. Wherever you feel the better stretch, hold for fifteen to twenty seconds and repeat three times.

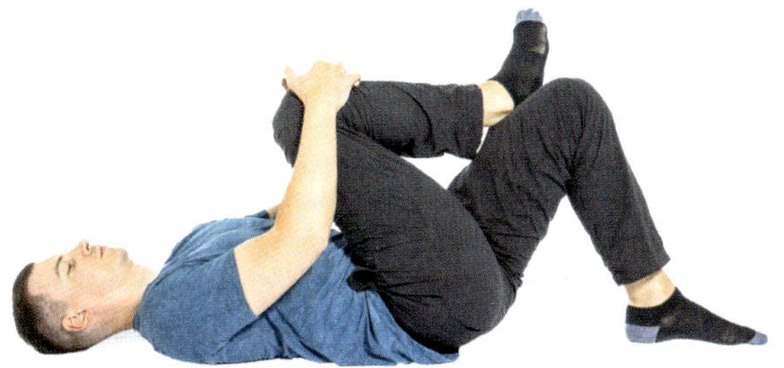

option 1

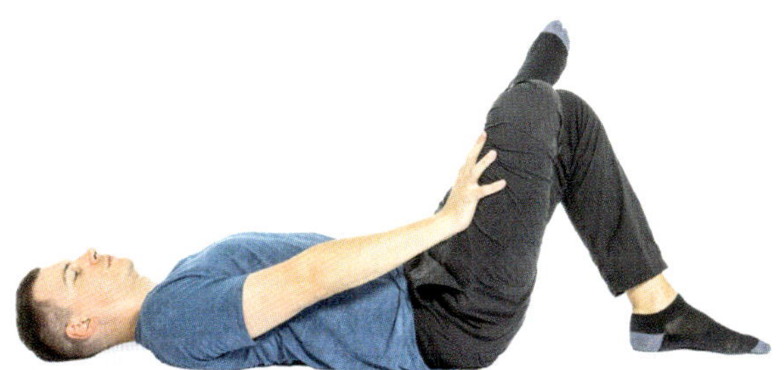

option 2

STRENGTHENING

LONG ARC QUAD ISOMETRIC HOLD (QUAD STRENGTHENING)

Sitting with both feet flat on the ground, and place an ankle weight on one ankle. Start with a fairly light weight, around three to five pounds, and make sure you can do the full number of reps and sets before adding weight. Straighten that leg and point your toes toward your face, really trying to use the quad as much as possible. Hold for forty-five seconds and repeat ten times, or hold for twenty-two seconds and repeat twenty times. Make sure that all you feel is the quad working and getting fatigued and no increase in pain in the knee.

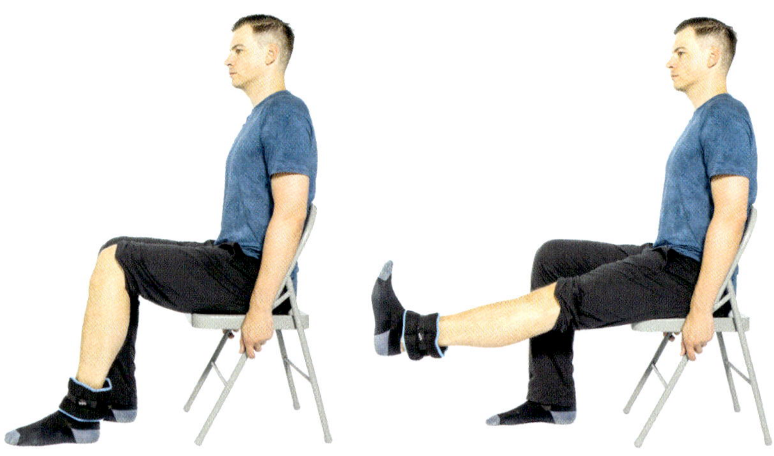

TERMINAL KNEE EXTENSIONS (TKES) (QUAD STRENGTHENING)

Secure one end of a resistance band out in front of you and loop the other end of the band behind your knee. Walk back far enough to create tension through the band with your knee slightly bent. Then fully straighten your knee, focusing on working the quad as much as possible. Hold for five seconds and repeat fifteen times.

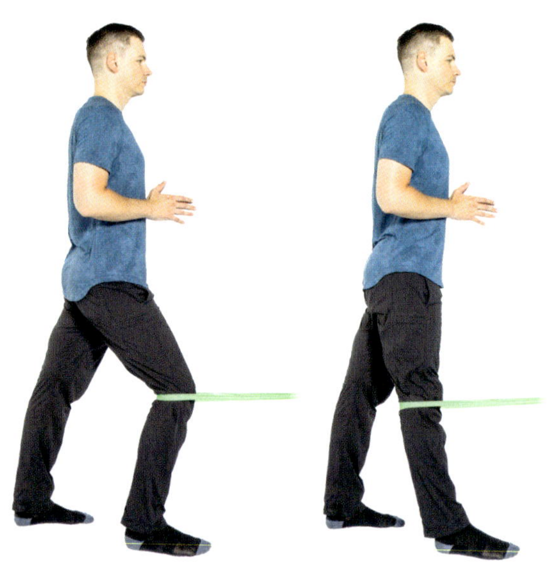

STEP-DOWNS (QUAD STRENGTHENING)

Standing on one leg, straighten the other leg out in front of you. On the standing leg, allow your knee to come forward as far as you can comfortably control it without leaning or turning. The goal is that you feel the quad working without increasing any pain in the knee. Once you've gone as far as you can, stand back up. Repeat this for two or three sets of ten.

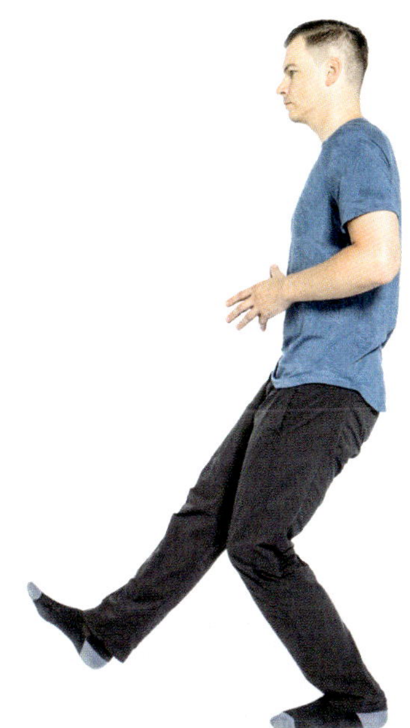

SINGLE-LEG RDLS (HAMSTRING/ GLUTE STRENGTHENING)

Stand with one leg out in front of you and the other leg behind you with the toe turned out. Bend the front knee slightly and keep all of your weight in your front heel. Cross your arms over your chest while keeping your chest tall and your back extended. Lean over at the waist until you feel a slight stretch in the back of the front leg, then squeeze your glute and stand back up to where you started. Repeat for two or three sets of ten. To make this exercise harder, simply hold some weights in your hands.

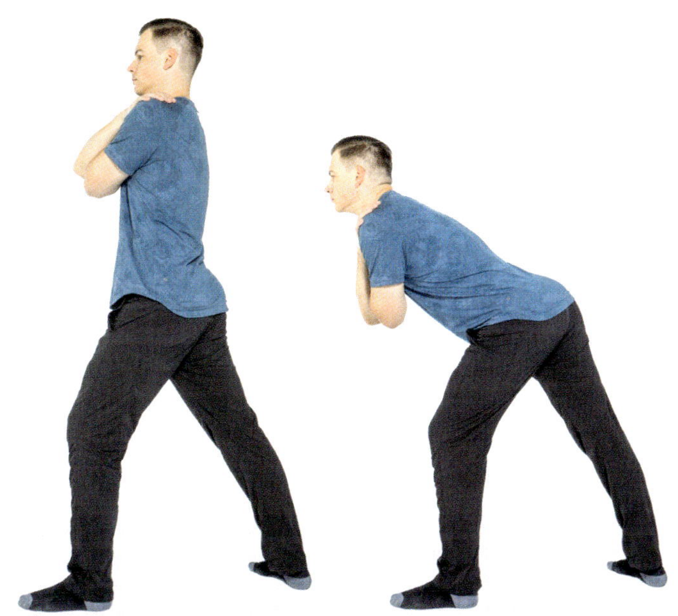

SINGLE-LEG ECCENTRIC BRIDGES (HAMSTRING/GLUTE STRENGTHENING)

Lying on your back with your knees bent, push through the floor using only your heels and lift your hips off the ground. At the top of the movement, lift one foot off the ground and lower your hips back down using only the leg on the ground. Do not twist or shift your weight, and move slowly and with control. Repeat for two or three sets of ten on each leg.

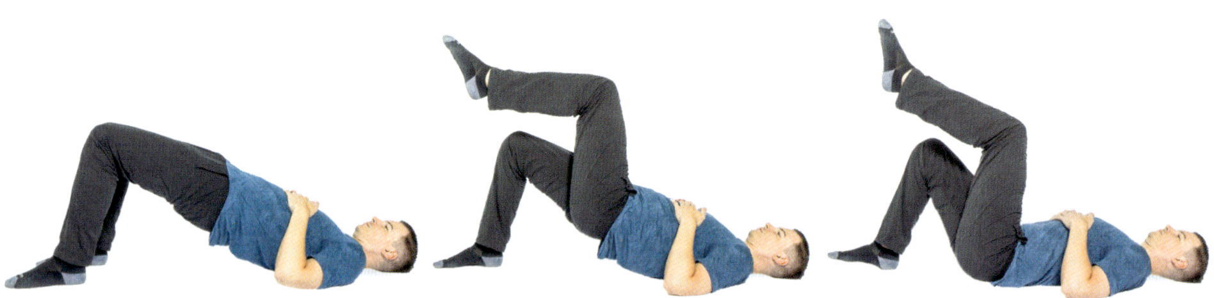

SEATED HIP FLEXION (HIP FLEXOR STRENGTHENING)

Seated on the ground, keep one knee bent with the other leg straight out in front of you. Place your hands on the bent knee and keep your chest tall and your lower back extended. Without leaning back or rounding your spine, lift the leg straight out in front of you off the ground as much as you can, then slowly lower it back to the ground. Repeat for two or three sets of ten on each leg.

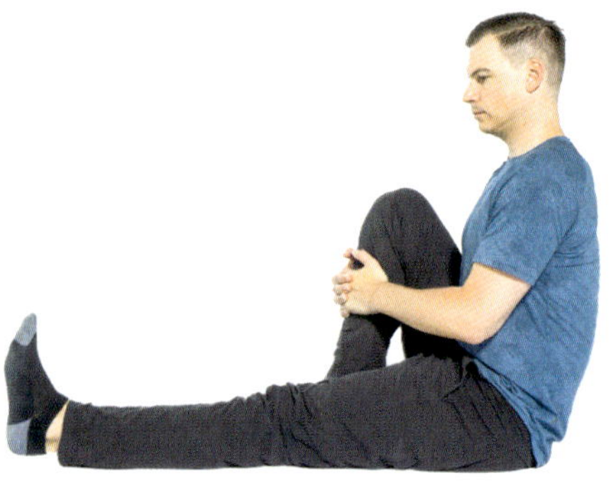

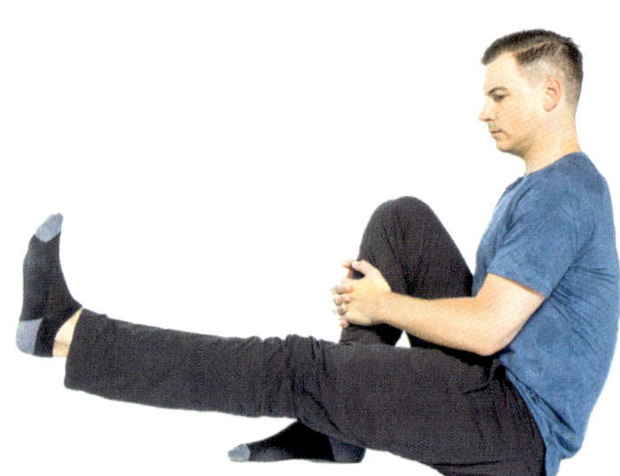

STRAIGHT-LEG RAISE WITH INTERNAL ROTATION (HIP FLEXOR/TFL STRENGTHENING)

Lie on your back and keep one knee bent with the other leg straight out in front of you. Keep the straight leg as straight as you can while also keeping the whole leg turned in. Keeping the knee locked straight and the leg turned in, raise that leg off of the ground as far as you can control it, then slowly lower it back to the ground. Repeat for two or three sets of ten on each leg.

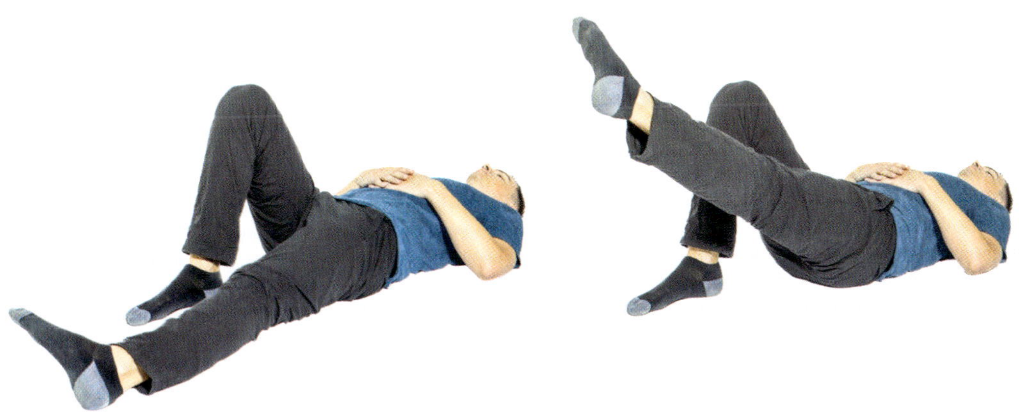

SIDE-LYING HIP ABDUCTION (GLUTE/HIP ABDUCTOR STRENGTHENING)

Lie on your side with the bottom leg bent and the top leg straight. Keep your top hip slightly forward and the top leg turned in. Without rolling your hip backward, keep the top leg straight and turned in as you raise it straight up toward the ceiling as far as you can control, then slowly lower it back down. Repeat for two or three sets of ten on each side.

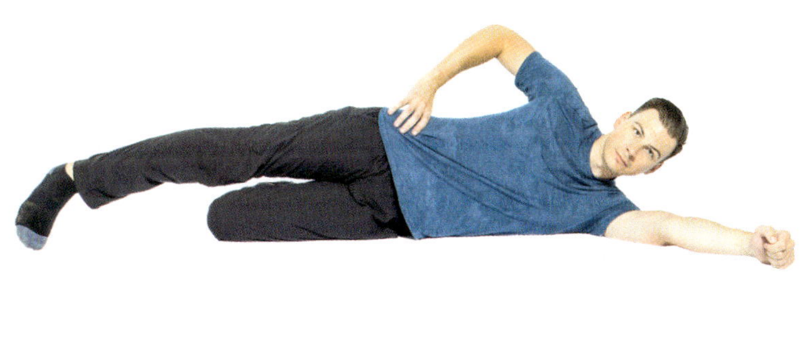

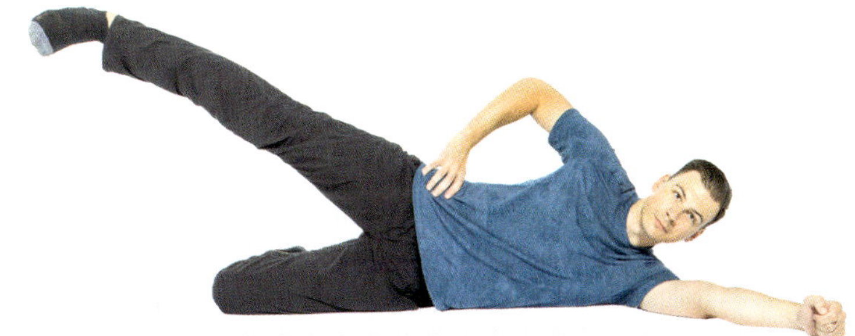

ELEVATED CLAMSHELLS (GLUTE/HIP ABDUCTOR STRENGTHENING)

Lie on your side with your knees bent and your feet elevated off the ground. Maintain a straight line from your feet to your butt to your shoulders. While keeping your heels together, open the top knee like a book. Make sure that your top hip doesn't roll backward, and be sure to open that top leg as far as you absolutely can. Repeat for two or three sets of ten on each leg.

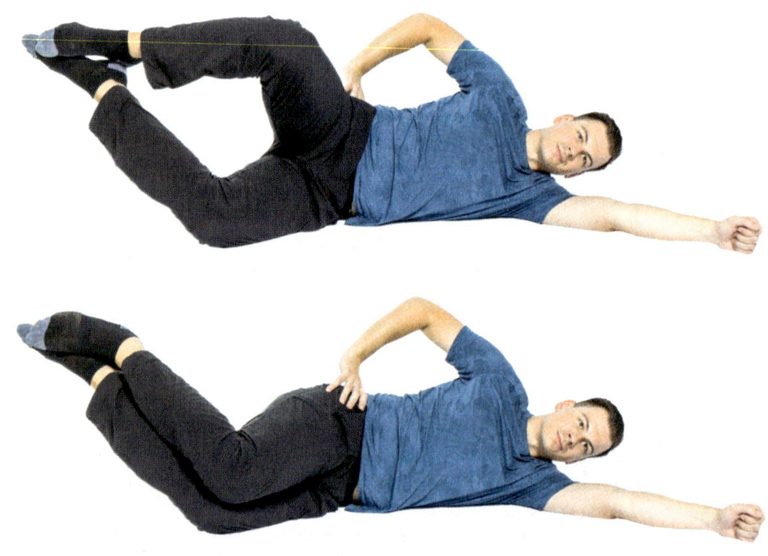

HIP ADDUCTION ISOMETRIC (HIP ADDUCTOR STRENGTHENING)

Lie on your back with your knees bent, and place a Pilates ring or small ball between your knees. Slowly bring your knees together, gradually building up the pressure you're using until you feel like you are really working your groin muscles without increasing your pain. Hold at that pressure for ten full seconds and repeat for two sets of ten.

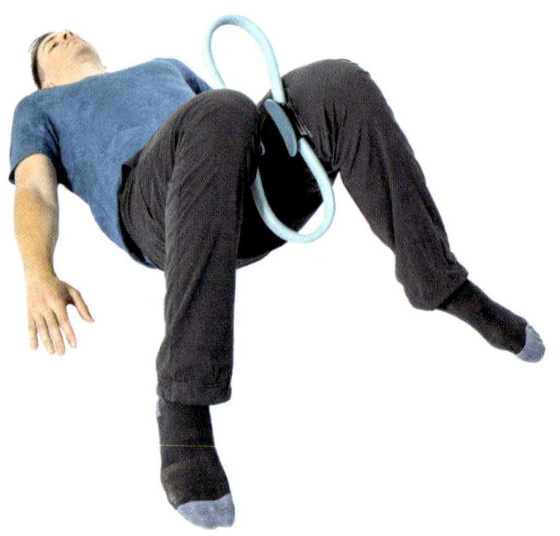

SECTION 3

THE LOWER BACK

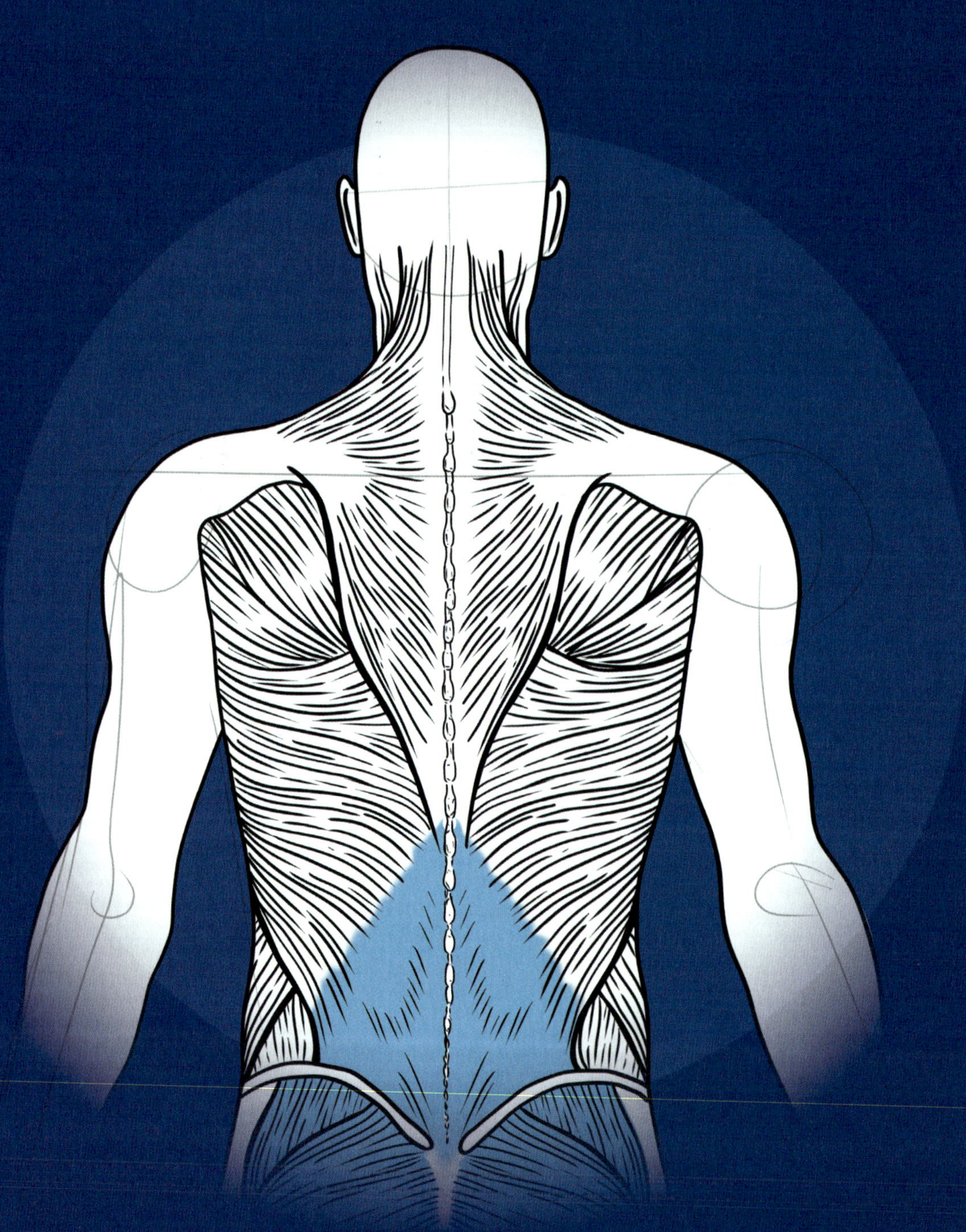

The lower back is possibly the most researched part of the body when it comes to the science of pain. There are whole books dedicated to it. When it came time for me to write about the lower back in this book, I knew there were a lot of ways I could have gone about it. The lower back is not only one of the most prevalent sources of pain but arguably also one of the most complex. A lot of different things can be going on in the lower back that can cause a wide array of symptoms. And a lot of times, the same exact problem can cause totally different symptoms in different people.

When getting an X-ray or MRI on the lower back, there is no guarantee that what your doctor sees is actually the source of your symptoms. Joints, bones, muscles, nerves, and discs can all present as causes of pain, and all of them can be the main culprit. Often, what looks the worst on an X-ray or MRI is not the cause of symptoms. In the lower back specifically, there is a relatively low correlation between what "looks the worst" on an image and what is causing the most pain. That uncertainty is a big reason why the outcomes of lower back surgeries can be so poor.

But for the same reasons that it is so complicated, pain in the lower back can be incredibly easy to deal with if you start with some simple steps. Since there are so many different things that could be wrong and so many ways that people feel symptoms, while it might seem counterintuitive, you must start with something uncomplicated, or you might never get a chance to start at all.

When I see a lower back pain patient in the clinic for the first time, I place their symptoms in one of three buckets that will determine what sort of advice and movements they receive to get started:

- **Bucket 1:** Pain that worsens primarily with rounding the lower back, such as bending over or sitting
- **Bucket 2:** Pain that worsens primarily with extending the lower back, such as leaning backward or standing
- **Bucket 3:** Pain that worsens with both rounding and extending, or a lower back that is just kind of painful all the time

Once I identify which of these three buckets a patient's pain falls into, I know the best way to start reducing symptoms. Once symptoms reduce and the patient becomes more confident in their ability to use the hip and core musculature, then they can progress to more challenging exercises and hopefully fully return to their normal lives pain free.

ANATOMY

The spine is split up into four main regions from top to bottom: cervical, thoracic, lumbar, and sacrum. The lower back comprises five lumbar vertebrae (the vertebrae are the bones that make up the spine). Your spinal cord runs through a hole in each vertebra, and in between each pair of vertebrae is a disc that provides cushioning between the bones. In between each spinal segment, you also have nerves that leave the spinal cord and extend throughout the body. Along with bones, discs, and nerves, you also have a variety of muscles in the lumbar spine. This beautiful, complicated mess has become the bane of many people's existences.

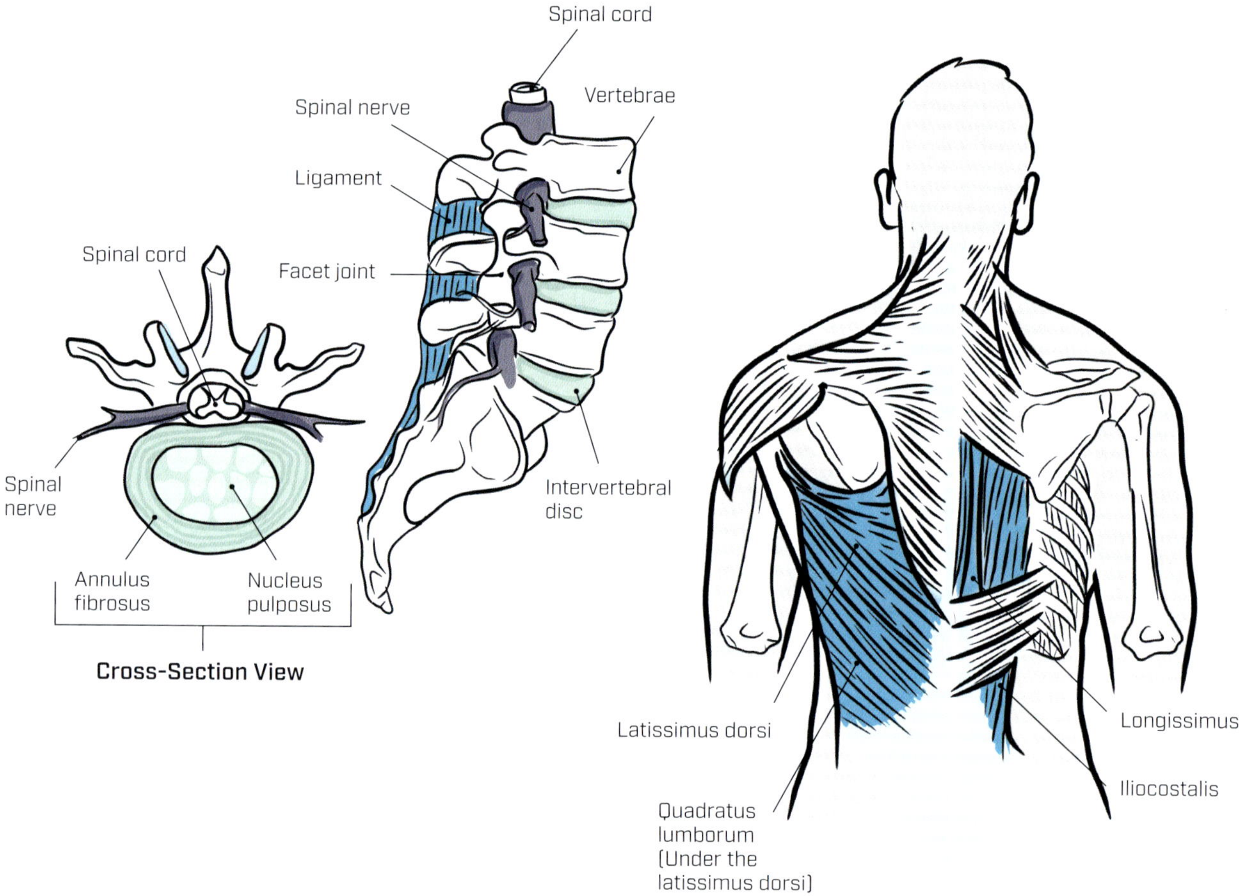

There are a lot of other small intricacies in the lower back, but since we are keeping this section simple, if you can just understand the bare bones (no pun intended) of the lower back as shown in the illustration, you're already way ahead of the game.

DERMATOME MAP

How the lower back can cause pain farther down the leg and sometimes all the way into the toes is best explained by something known as a dermatome map.

The dermatome map shows where in your legs you will feel nerve pain based on where that nerve is being irritated in the lower back. On the map, you will see certain areas highlighted and labeled with a different lumbar segment. For instance, the nerves that control feeling in the L1 section are the nerves that come out below the first lumbar vertebra (L1). The section labeled L2 is the nerves that come out below the second lumbar vertebra, and so on. The sections labeled with "S" follow the same rules but come from the region just below the lumbar region, the sacrum.

Most people who experience nerve pain feel it very specifically in one or two of these regions, and that is how you can find out where in the lower back pain is coming from. In general, the farther away you feel pain from the actual source, the more irritation there is back at the root. For instance, the L5 nerve root controls sensation along the outside of the leg and down to the foot. If you feel nerve pain all the way down into the foot, there is likely more irritation present than there is for someone who only feels nerve pain in the side of the leg.

Where exactly the nerve pain is coming from doesn't make a big difference in terms of which bucket you fall into or what exercises you will end up doing. But I have always felt that this was an important thing to understand when trying to grasp the overall anatomy of the lower back and how nerve pain can happen.

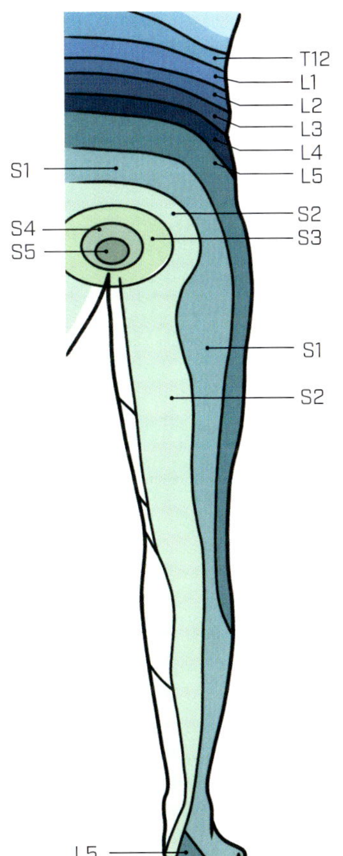

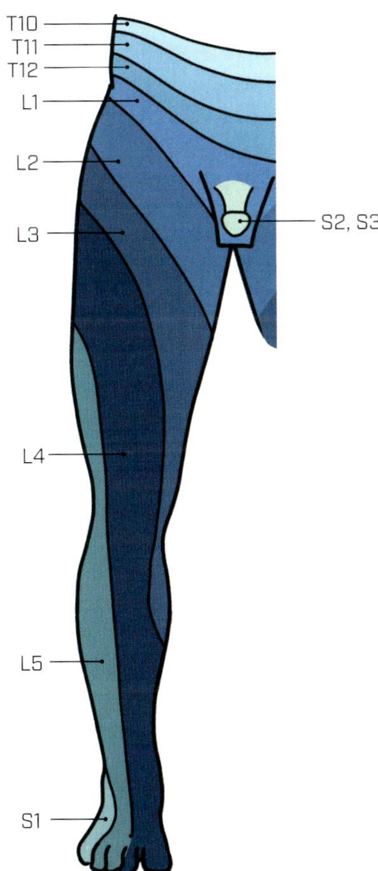

BUCKET 1: PAIN WHEN ROUNDING THE LOWER BACK

If you find that your lower back pain reliably gets worse when you do things like bend at the waist, sit for a prolonged period of time, lift a heavy object, or reach out in front of you, then you are firmly in bucket number one. And when you are firmly in this bucket, there is a good chance that the primary source of your pain is one of the discs in your lower back. Especially if this pain started after you lifted a heavy object or gets worse with things like coughing and sneezing, then the disc is your likely culprit.

Disc injuries can sound scary, but almost all of us know someone who has had a herniated disc or maybe even had surgery on a disc. Once you understand exactly what the disc is, how it operates, and how it causes pain, it becomes a lot less intimidating.

The anatomy of the disc is most commonly described as a jelly donut. The "jelly" is a thick fluid-like material called the nucleus pulposus that sits inside the disc, and the "doughnut" portion is a ligament called the annulus fibrosus that keeps the jelly in place.

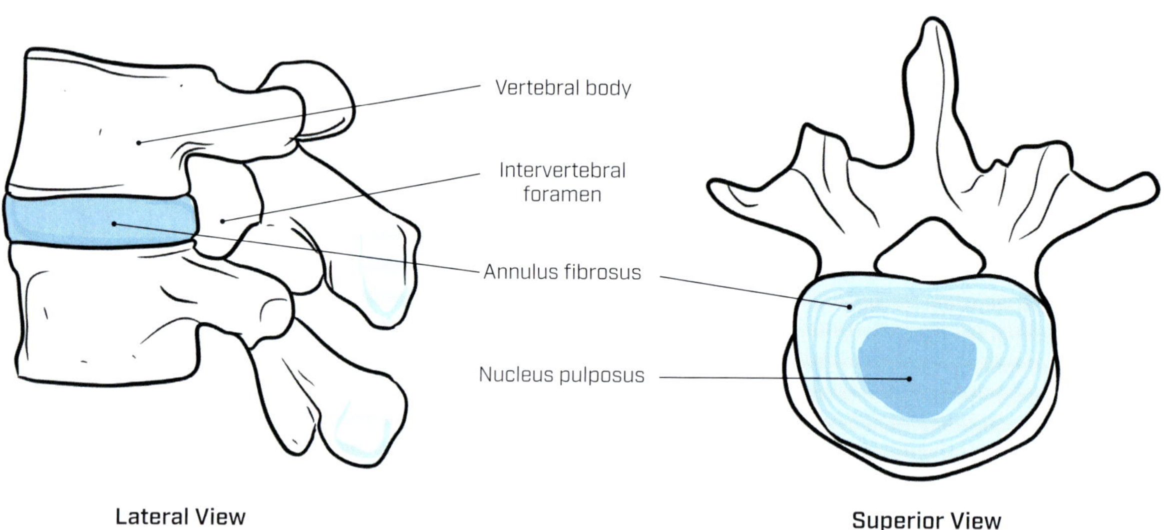

Lateral View

Superior View

When you injure a disc, you most commonly injure the back wall of the disc. When you lean forward or round your lower back, you push the jelly inside the disc toward the back wall. And when you create enough pressure on the back wall, you can sprain that ligament, and the jelly will be able to push out the back enough to press on the nerves in the area and create pain.

Technically speaking, the disc is only herniated once it creates a hole in the back wall and the jelly leaves the disc itself. In the grand scheme of disc injuries, this is pretty rare, despite plenty of MDs and practitioners labeling any disc injury as a "herniation." The much more common presentation is disc bulging, as shown in the illustration. The fact that the ligament is just sprained and the disc is just bulging is why these injuries respond so well to physical therapy.

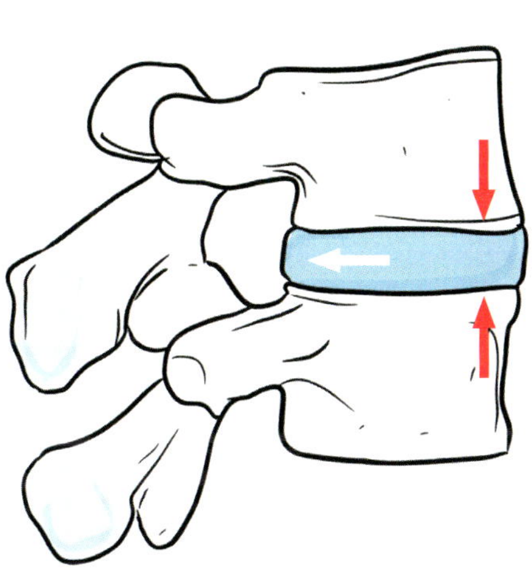

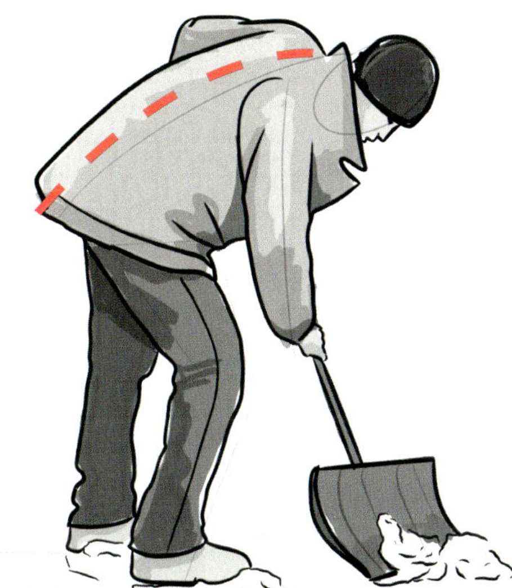

The main reason lumbar disc injuries can be so stubborn is that so many people spend most of their days sitting with a rounded lower back posture. Continuing to place pressure on a disc with an injury to the back wall is the equivalent of constantly poking a bruise and not allowing it to heal.

Think about it like this: When you sprain your ankle, the ankle can feel a little loose for a couple of weeks, and you may feel like you are always one small misstep away from irritating the injury again. But if you protect the ankle by placing it in a brace and walking carefully, you can allow that ligament to heal and become strong and stable again. Spraining your ankle and then spending eight to ten hours a day putting pressure on it is the same thing as having a disc injury and spending eight to ten hours a day sitting with a rounded lower back.

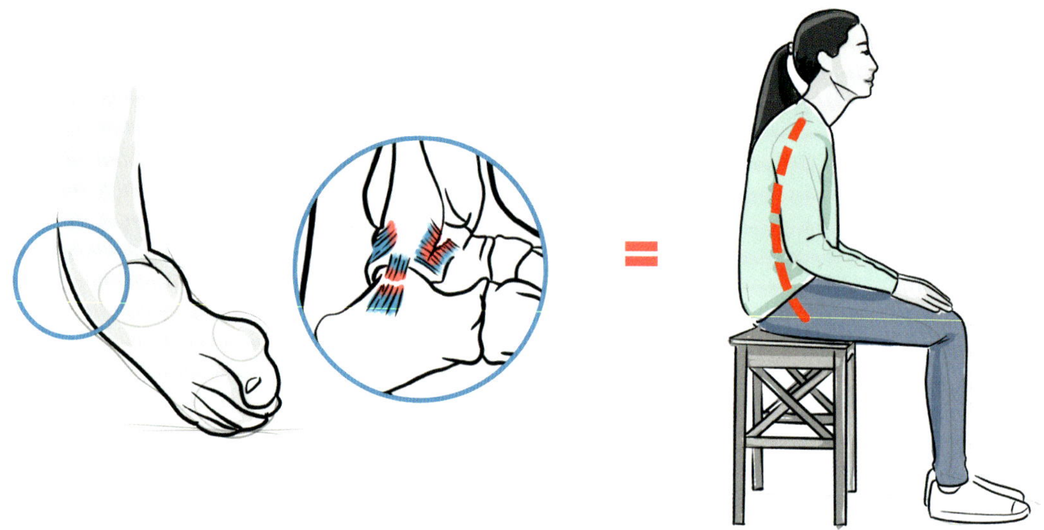

So, when you are in this bucket, the most important thing you can do is limit how often you have a rounded lower back. Stop doing any action that causes rounding of the lower back, such as stretching forward or bending over toward the ground. If you are sitting, make sure that you keep a rolled-up towel or lumbar support behind your lower back to prevent it from rounding. And, as much as possible, spend time either standing or lying on your stomach. The more time you can spend without rounding the lower back, the quicker the back wall of the disc can heal and stiffen back up.

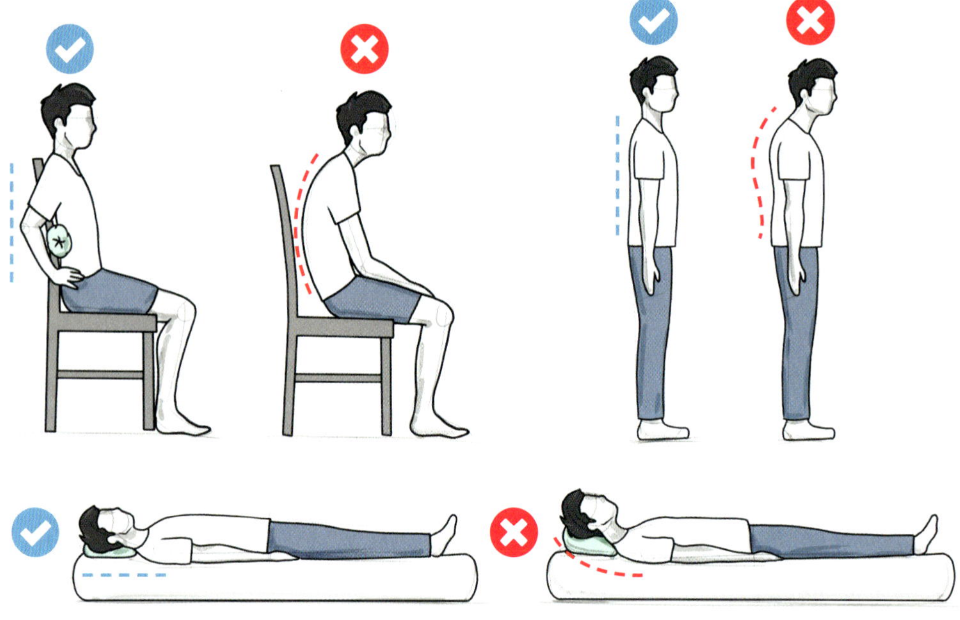

Every time your lower back starts to round, alarm bells should be going off in your head reminding you to straighten back up. Whenever you have an injury to the disc or the lower back in general, the muscles of the lower back will be tight. So, in the short term, stretches like child's pose or downward dog may feel okay, but in the long term, they will only delay the healing process. The goal is that after a few weeks of focusing on not rounding and practicing the two movements listed next, you will feel a massive difference in your symptoms. As symptoms start to subside and you feel more comfortable, you can also start doing the exercises starting on page 106.

Finally, it's important to note that this aversion to rounding the lower back should not be a lifelong sentence. Once the injury heals, it's actually a good idea to start slowly building your tolerance to rounding back up. Bending at the lower back is a very practical and functional skill; it's just something that can't be rushed in the presence of a disc injury.

MOVEMENTS TO REDUCE SYMPTOMS

PRONE LYING

As mentioned previously, lying on your stomach is one of the best positions because you can keep your lower back slightly extended while also keeping it completely supported and relaxed. It's by far the easiest exercise in this book. Simply lie on your stomach propped up on your elbows and stay there for ten to twenty minutes a few times a day. You can even read a book or scroll on your phone while you're doing it.

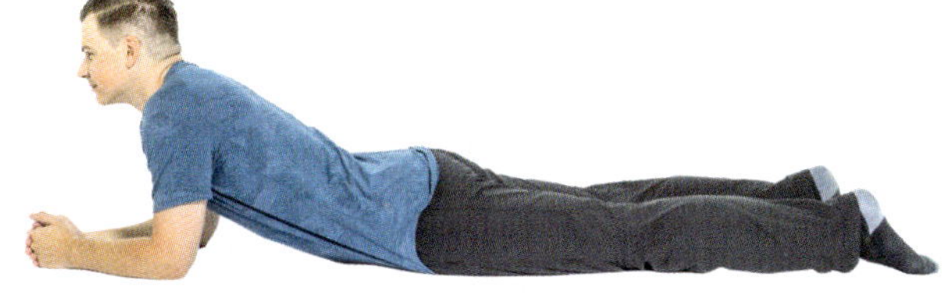

PRONE PRESS-UP

After doing some prone lying, you can follow it up with some prone press-ups. Place your hands underneath your shoulders like you're about to do a push-up. Focus on keeping everything below your shoulder blades completely relaxed as you push your chest off the floor until you feel a gentle pressure in your lower back. Hold for about a second and then lower yourself back down. Repeat for two sets of ten, two or three times per day.

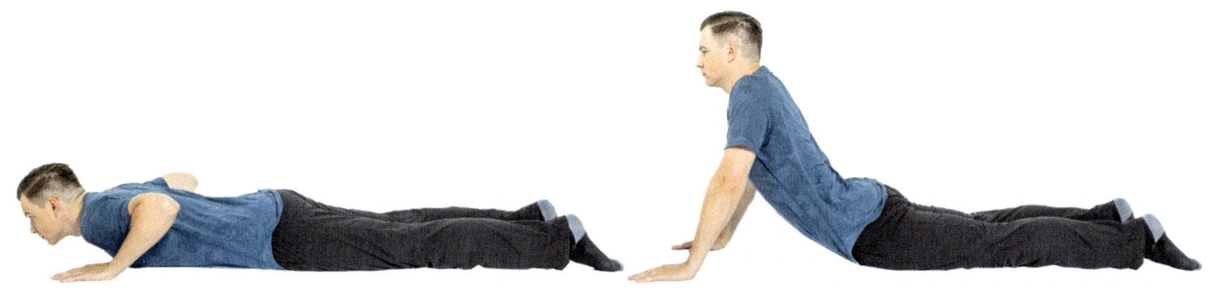

Both of these movements are meant to reduce your symptoms. If you find that they cause discomfort, try doing them for less time or with less extension in your lower back. For instance, if doing the prone lying while propped up on your elbows is too much, then just lie flat on your stomach. If you find that fifteen minutes is bothersome, try doing it for just five minutes. Once you find the modification that allows you to feel a reduction in symptoms afterward, stay there and build up slowly.

If you have a disc injury, these movements will not make anything worse, but if there is a lot of swelling and irritation in the area, they may be uncomfortable at first.

BUCKET 2: PAIN WITH EXTENDING THE LOWER BACK

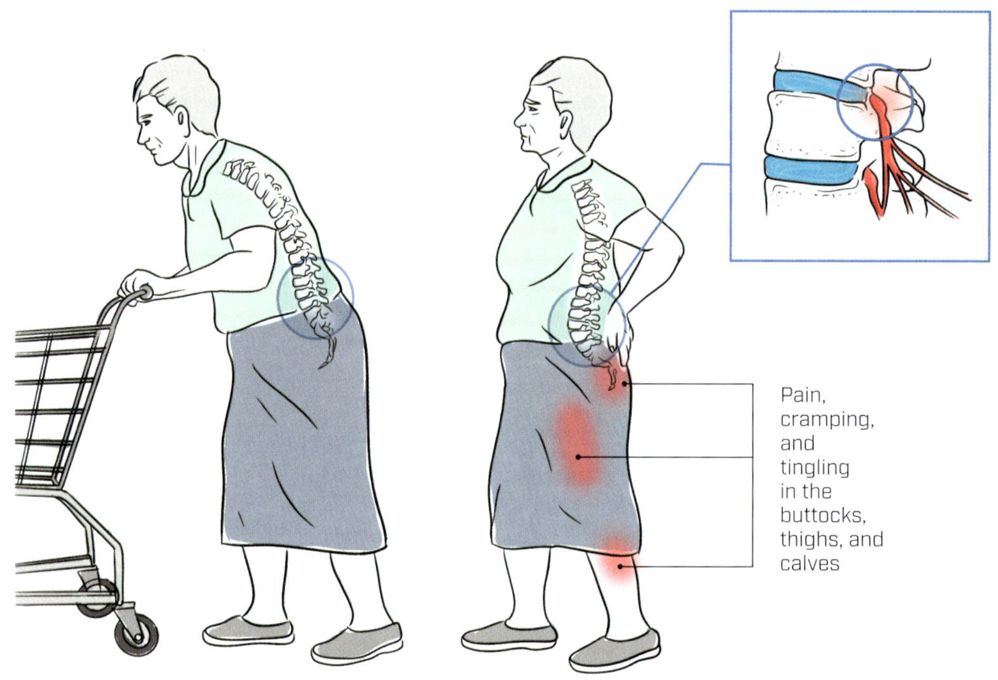

If your pain reliably gets worse when standing for prolonged periods of time, lying on your stomach, or leaning backward, then you are in this bucket. Also, if you have received a diagnosis such as arthritis, stenosis, degenerative disc disease (DDD), or spondylolisthesis, among others, then you are in this bucket. While the pain associated with rounding the lower back is almost always tied to the disc, pain that increases when moving the back in the opposite direction is almost always tied to the bones and joints of the lower back. All of the diagnoses I just listed cause inflammation in the joints or reduce the space between the joints. And when you extend your lower back, you bring those bones closer together and compress the joints, which increases pain.

With arthritis, stenosis, and DDD, space between the vertebrae can reduce enough that when extending your lower back, the joints clamp down on the nerve roots where they exit the spinal canal and cause referred pain down the leg. If you find that the longer you are on your feet, a certain part of your leg becomes numb or painful, this is most likely what you are dealing with. If you are interested in exactly where this nerve impingement is happening, refer to the dermatome map on page 97 and trace where you feel your discomfort back to its specific nerve root.

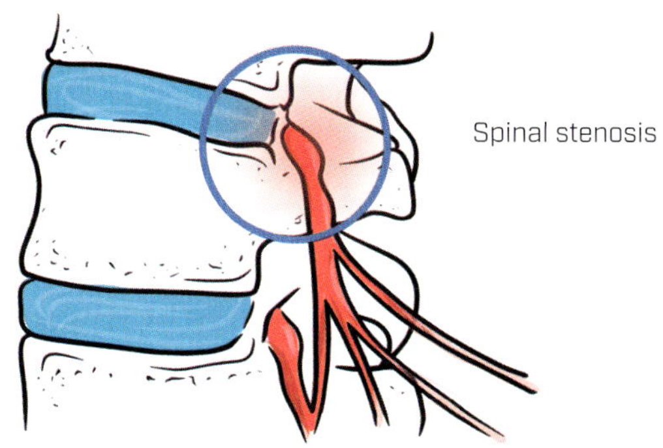
Spinal stenosis

Since extending the lower back increases in pain, rounding the lower back is the best way to bring some relief, which is why the suggested movements on page 104 put the back in that position. It is also a good idea to avoid activities that worsen this pain. So, limiting time spent on your feet or lying on your stomach is a good idea. As you spend less time in extension, the irritation in your lumbar vertebrae will start to calm down. Even though there is nothing you can do to reverse the process of something like arthritis, stenosis, or DDD, you can certainly reduce symptoms by avoiding extension for a period of time. A lot of people even find that if they can get the irritation to go down, extending the lower back becomes a lot more comfortable. That's because a lot of the discomfort wasn't coming from "bone on bone" compression; it was coming from swelling and irritation in the area.

As your symptoms start to decrease, it is a good idea to do the exercises starting on page 106 to start to build as much strength and control as possible so that your muscles can support you instead of the spine itself. The more work the spine has to do, the quicker your injury will become irritated and the more symptoms you will experience. But if you can take weight off your spine by making your muscles do the work, you will find that you can do so much more without an increase in pain.

MOVEMENTS TO REDUCE SYMPTOMS

SINGLE KNEE TO CHEST

Lying on your back with your knees bent, take one knee in both hands and bring it toward your chest. The goal is to feel a gentle stretch in your lower back on the side of the leg you are holding. If you feel a pressure in the front of your hip as you bring your knee up, try keeping your knee more toward the outside of your body. Once you feel a stretch, hold for twenty to thirty seconds and repeat three times on each leg. Feel free to do this exercise multiple times per day.

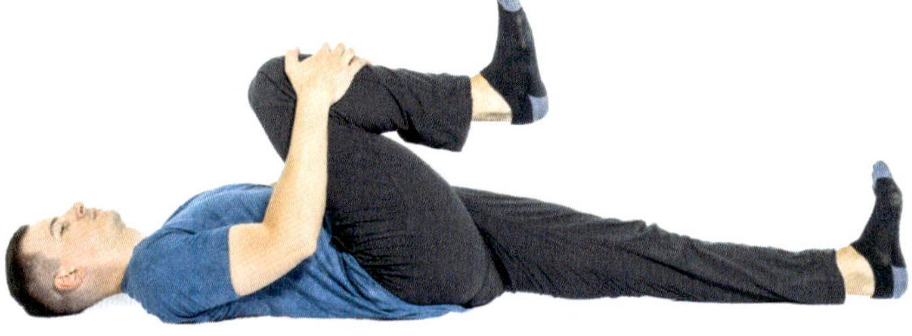

SEATED REACH

Sitting in a chair with a table in front of you and your legs spread apart, reach forward. Place your palms on the table and continue to reach forward without rising up from the chair. Once you feel a small stretch in your lower back, hold for fifteen to twenty seconds and repeat three times. You can try moving your hands to one side or the other to see if you can find a better stretch. Repeat as needed throughout the day.

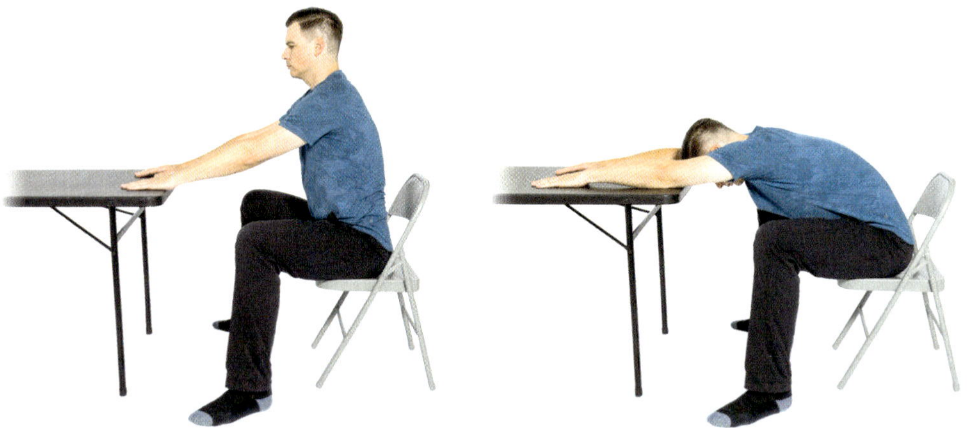

These movements are meant to reduce your symptoms. If you find that they worsen your symptoms, try not to push them as far, and make sure what you're feeling is gentle. If they are still worsening your symptoms, read the other two buckets to make sure you're following the advice that applies most directly to you.

BUCKET 3: PAIN WITH BOTH ROUNDING AND EXTENDING THE LOWER BACK

Welcome to the dreaded "pain with everything" bucket. If you're in this bucket, you may have a combination of disc-related pain and joint-related pain. Since you're experiencing both issues, there is no reliable way to reduce symptoms with certain positions. And it may seem like any position you get in ultimately leads to pain. This may also be the case if you have a strained or irritated muscle in your lower back. Since that muscle is active every time you move in a different direction, it can feel like it is always irritated. Another cause of winding up in this bucket is general instability of the spine.

If you do have a combination of a disc issue and a joint issue, none of the symptom-reducing movements listed in those first two buckets will do you much good, so it's a good idea to jump straight to the strengthening exercises starting on page 106. As you improve the strength of your hips and core, you will take a lot of stress away from your lower back, and that reduction in stress will result in a reduction in symptoms.

If you have a muscular issue in your lower back, it is still a good idea to jump straight to the strengthening exercises for two main reasons:

1. The muscle may be tight only because of irritation in the lower back that is being caused by either a disc issue or a joint issue. And since the muscular tightness may be masking the true cause, you don't want to commit to either type of symptom-reducing movement. The symptom-reducing movements in one bucket are exactly what increase symptoms in the other bucket. That is exactly why I almost never give someone stretches for muscle pain in the lower back.
2. The muscles in the lower back are probably only tight or strained because the muscles in the core and hips aren't strong enough. And when you aren't getting enough strength from your core and hips, the muscles of your lower back begin to take over. This often results in the lower back muscles taking on too much and getting strained as a result. Therefore, jumping straight to the exercises for the core and the hips is the best way to address the true cause of the pain.

If you have general instability of the spine, you may feel an increase in pain with every movement. Since I work with a lot of very flexible people, like dancers, this is something I see quite often. The more flexible and mobile somebody is, the more important it becomes to be strong and stable through the muscles of the core and the hips. Especially if you are both flexible and mobile and doing something like dancing or some other form of physically taxing movement, you need to provide your spine with as much muscular strength as possible. If you're lacking the strength required to control the mobility of the spine, your joints will be constantly irritated and will land you squarely in this bucket.

A condition like scoliosis can also land you in this bucket. Scoliosis is a common diagnosis for a slight curve in the spine. It should be tracked over time by a practitioner, and if the curve gets big enough, a brace may be recommended. A lot of people have a small scoliosis curve that doesn't require formal attention but can cause a lot of muscular discomfort. Since there is a curve in the spine, the muscles can't work symmetrically as intended. Getting started with these exercises is a great idea because building strength and moving more will always help any sort of muscular discomfort. But it may be wise to see a professional to understand exactly where your particular asymmetries are depending on your curve.

STRENGTHENING MOVEMENTS FOR THE LOWER BACK

LEVEL ONE

Level one involves three exercises that are done with a Pilates ring. The name of the game for these three movements is core activation and muscle coordination, all while the back is in a supported and neutral position. For all of these exercises, the goal is to feel the muscles working without any increase in pain or tightness in the lower back. Once you can do these three exercises comfortably on a daily basis, you can progress to level two.

PILATES RING CORE BRACING

Lying on your back with your knees bent, place one end of the Pilates ring on your thighs and stabilize the other end with your hands, keeping your arms straight. Brace your stomach as if a bowling ball were going to fall from the ceiling and land on your belly button. Press into the ring, and you should feel your core really kick on. Once you feel that sensation, hold for a long second and repeat for three sets of ten.

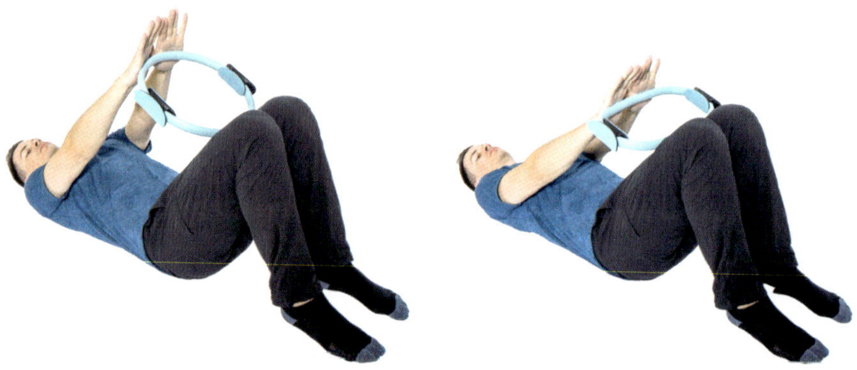

PILATES RING HIP ABDUCTION

Lying on your back with your knees bent, place the Pilates ring around your knees. Brace your core for the imaginary bowling ball, and press your knees out against the ring. As you do so, you should feel the muscles in the sides of your hips working. Once you feel that sensation, squeeze your glutes together. Ultimately, in the position you are holding for one long second, the core is braced, the knees are out, and the glutes are squeezed. Repeat for three sets of ten.

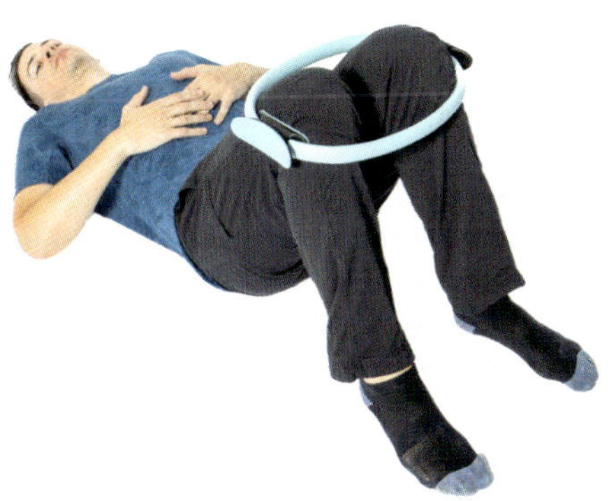

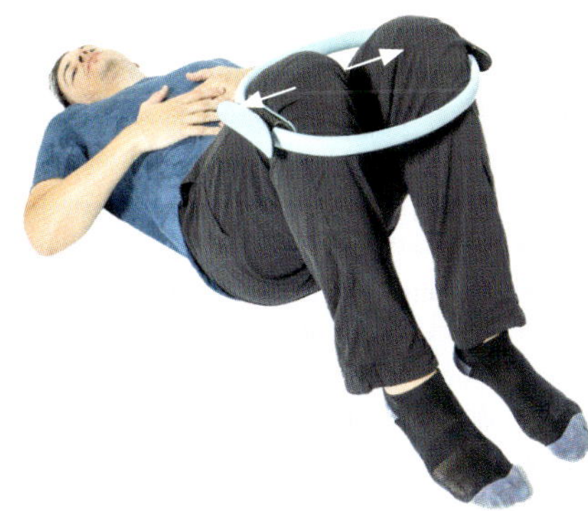

PILATES RING HIP ADDUCTION

Lying on your back with your knees bent, place the Pilates ring between your knees. Brace your core for the imaginary bowling ball and press your knees together against the ring until you feel your groin muscles activate. Once you feel that, keep your core braced and hold for one long second. Repeat for three sets of ten.

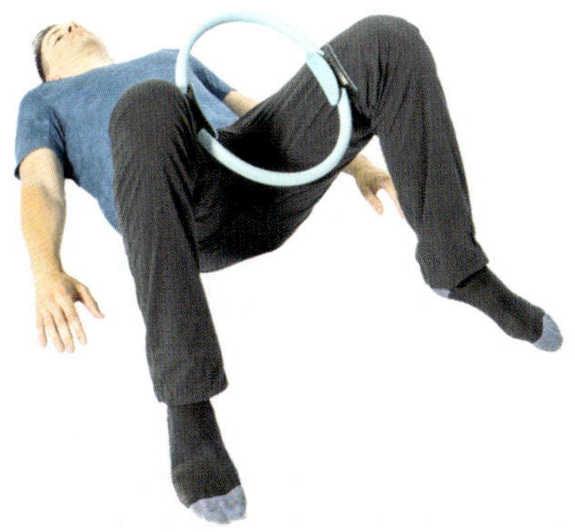

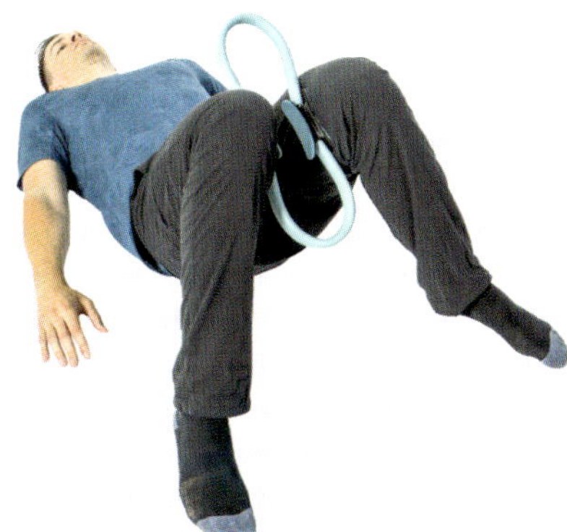

LEVEL TWO

Start by doing the exercises from level one as a warm-up. Just as in level one, you want to be able to do these exercises on a daily basis without feeling any increase in pain or discomfort in the lower back before moving on to level three.

DEAD BUGS

Lying on your back, stick your arms straight up toward the ceiling and raise your legs, keeping your hips and knees at 90-degree angles. Brace your core for the imaginary bowling ball and extend one arm and the opposite leg down toward the floor as far as you can comfortably control. Make sure that you can do this movement without your lower back moving and without feeling any discomfort. As you get more comfortable with the movement, you can begin to extend your arm and leg closer to the ground, but you don't want to rush the process. Once you find a comfortable range, repeat for two sets of ten on each side.

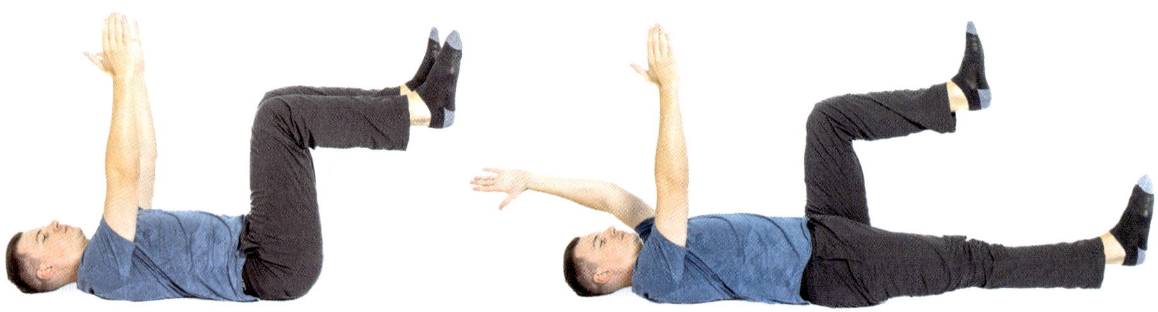

KNEELING SIDE PLANKS

On a yoga mat or carpeted floor, or using some form of cushion for your knees and elbows, rise up into a kneeling side plank, trying to maintain a straight line from your knees to your glutes to your shoulders. While holding the side plank, you should feel the side of your abs and the side of your hips that are closest to the floor activating. Hold for fifteen to twenty seconds and repeat three times on each side.

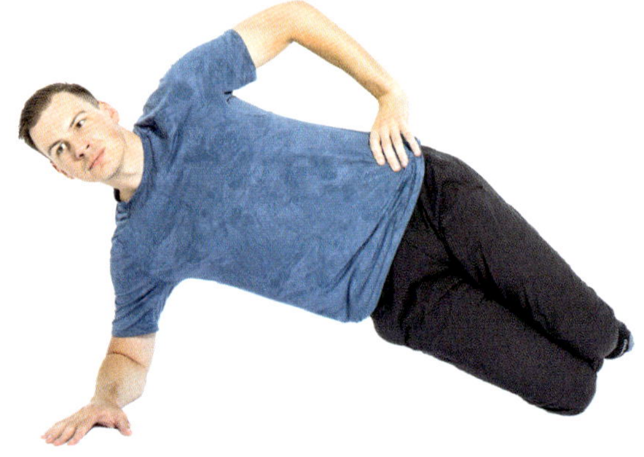

BIRD DOGS

Use the same form of cushion that you used for the side planks for this exercise. Position yourself on your hands and knees, maintain a neutral spine, and keep your core braced for the imaginary bowling ball. Without twisting or leaning one way or the other, extend one arm in front of you while extending the opposite leg behind you. This is basically the same movement as the dead bug, but it is more difficult because your back isn't being supported. Repeat for three sets of ten on each side.

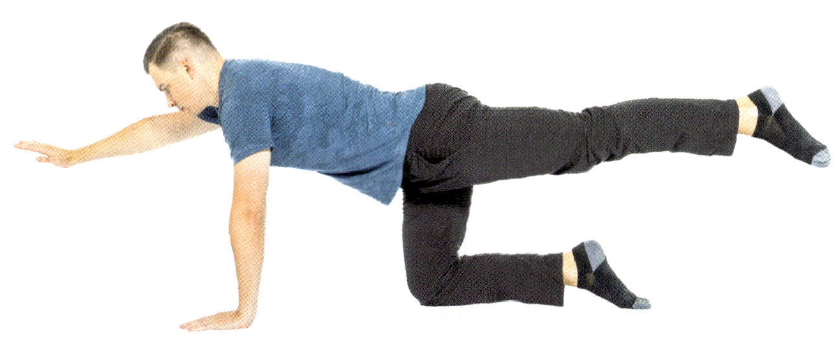

LEVEL THREE

This level is truly what you make of it. I'm a big believer that the best form of exercise is the exercise that you enjoy doing, because the exercise that you enjoy doing is the one you are most likely to stick to on a consistent basis. For me, that involves lifting weights and resistance training. For others, it may be Pilates or yoga. No matter what it is, you want to do some form of exercise at least two to three days a week and ideally include some form of resistance training. Whether you use weights, resistance bands, or just your body weight (like the exercises in level two), resistance training is a tried-and-true way to stay strong and healthy as you age. So, if your regular form of exercise is cardio based, like walking or biking, it is important to keep up the exercises from level two in addition to that. If you are doing weightlifting or Pilates, remember the principles of these exercises. No matter what exercise you do, focus on keeping the core braced, the back neutral, and feeling the muscles of the abs and hips. If you can follow those key ideas, you should be able to do any exercise safely and without pain.

SECTION 4

THE MID BACK

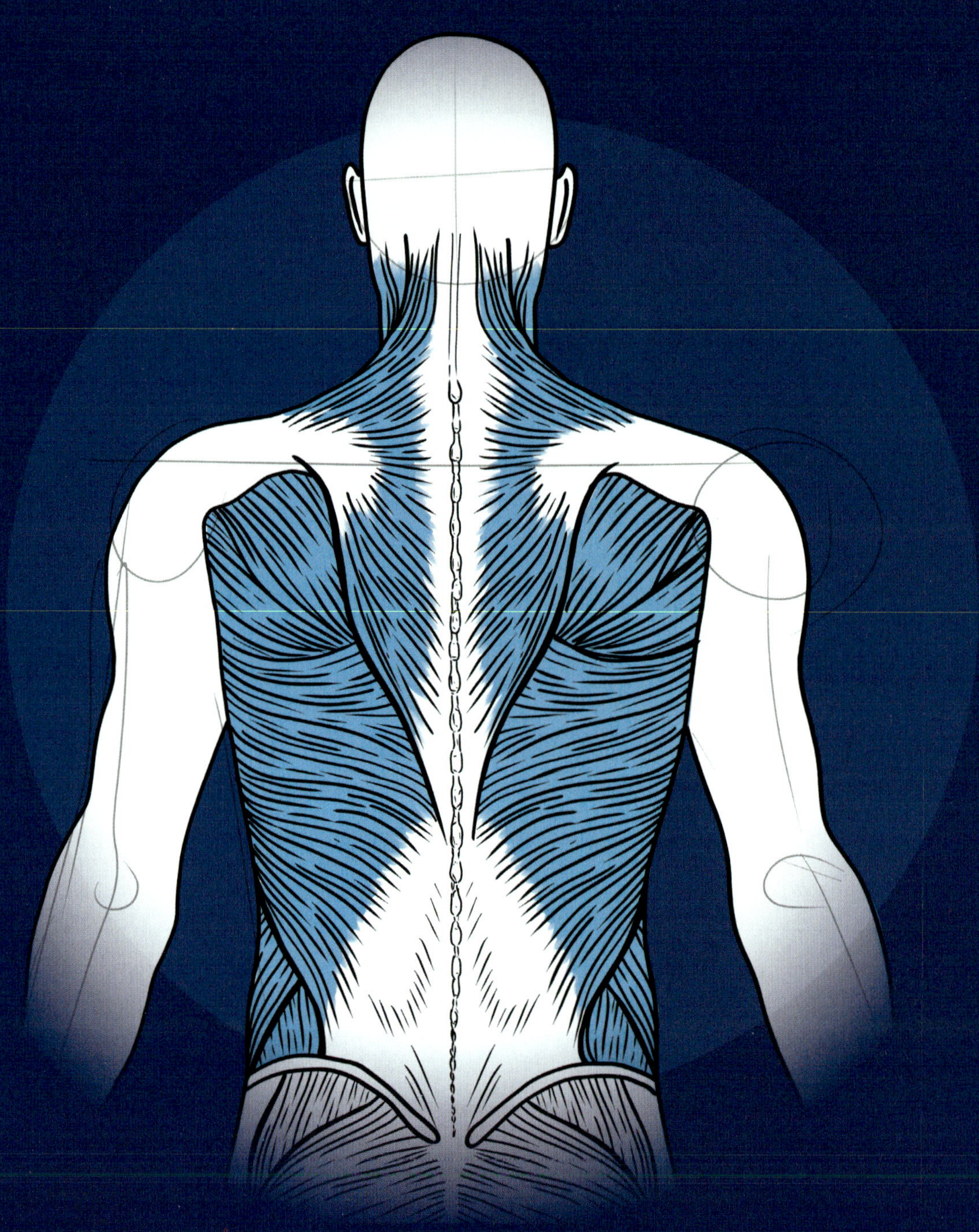

As mentioned in other parts of this book, the spine is made up of four main regions: the cervical, thoracic, lumbar, and sacrum. The mid back is comprised of the twelve vertebrae that make up the thoracic spine. The vertebrae in the thoracic region differ greatly from the ones found in other regions. These vertebrae are built in a way that makes it tough for them to bend and extend, but they're very good at rotating. That's why you feel like most of the bending and extending in the spine comes from the neck and the lower back.

There is also one huge and noticeable difference in the thoracic vertebrae: Each one has a rib coming out of either end. Your first rib comes out of the first thoracic vertebra, and your twelfth and final rib comes out of your twelfth and final thoracic vertebra. The thoracic region is also where the shoulder blades and a lot of important musculature lie. The muscles on the shoulder blade will be addressed in the shoulder section starting on page 141. This section just covers the musculature that surrounds them.

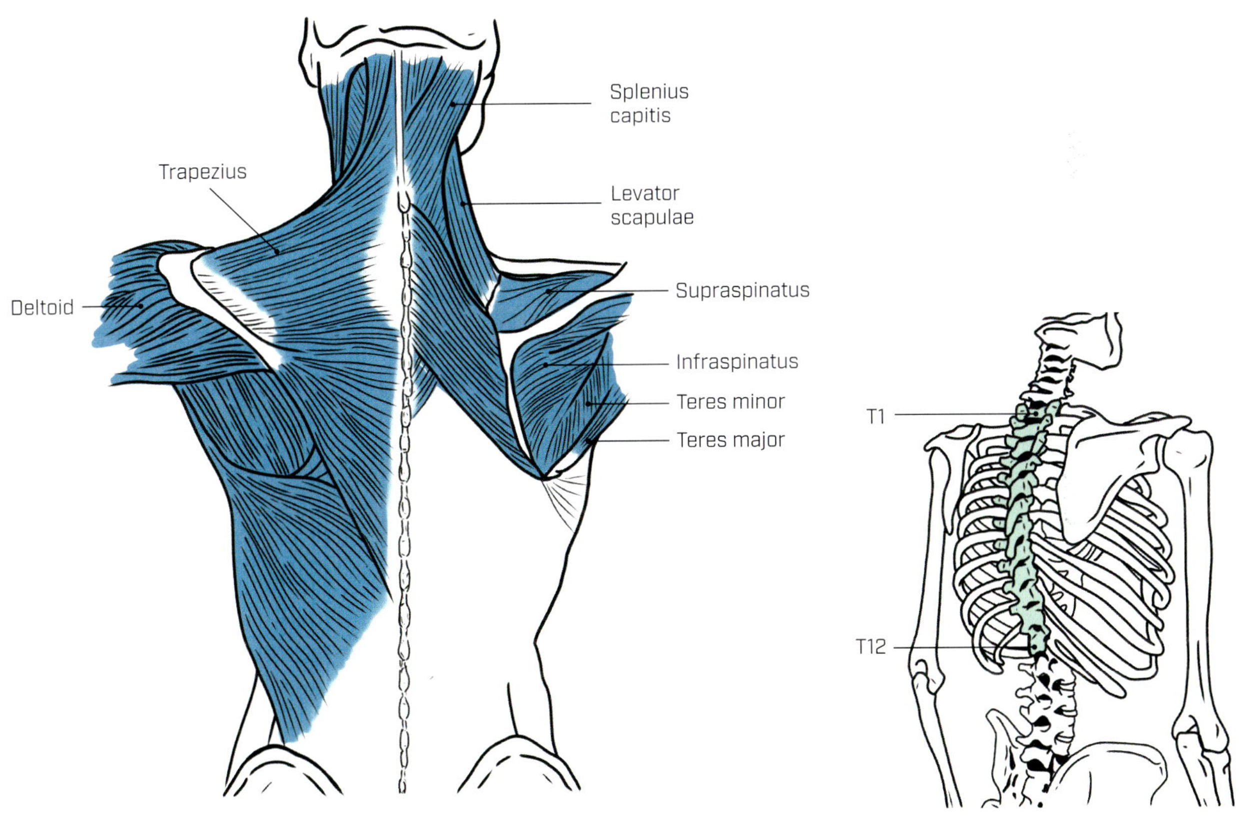

The mid back is a common source of pain, tightness, and postural insecurities, especially in people who work at a desk or have a crippling phone addiction. But with just a little bit of knowledge about the thoracic spine and by integrating some simple movements, you can make a very big difference fairly quickly.

DOWAGER'S HUMP, THORACIC KYPHOSIS, AND BUFFALO HUMP

Dowager's hump and excessive thoracic kyphosis are essentially the same thing: The mid and upper back are more rounded than they should be. Everyone has a natural level of kyphosis (*kyphosis* just means a rounding in the spine), meaning that a perfectly normal and healthy mid back has a slight round to it. But when that rounding becomes excessive, it can give the impression of a "hump." People who work at a desk or know that they spend too much time in a slouched position often fear that they will develop the diagnosis most commonly associated with great-grandparents and the Hunchback of Notre Dame. I have had patients so afraid of developing an upp-back hump that they have made appointments with me just to avoid it, even though they weren't in pain.

Buffalo hump is a medical condition that is commonly associated with Cushing's disease. When this is the case, the movements and exercises described here can make a slight difference and reduce discomfort, but there will likely always be some form of a hump present.

Normal Thoracic Kyphosis vs. Excessive Kyphosis

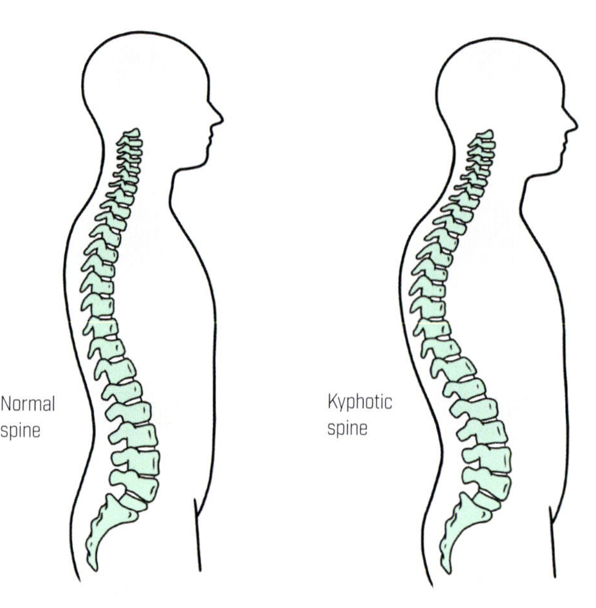

If your condition isn't buffalo hump and you would like to reverse it, the best place to start is with the thoracic mobilizations found on page 119. It is also important to work on the mid back–strengthening exercises found on page 121 and the rotator cuff exercises found on page 157. The mobilizations will make it easier to straighten the thoracic spine, and the exercises will help give you the strength to stay there.

Along with the mobilizations and exercises, it is important to avoid spending long periods of time in a slouched position. I normally suggest that every thirty to forty-five minutes, you stand up and at least move the mid back around a little bit, ideally by doing some of the mobilizations from this book. Breaking up your posture throughout the day will reduce the amount of tightness and rounding you feel in this area.

SCOLIOSIS

Another diagnosis that can cause a "hump" in the mid back is scoliosis. Scoliosis is when there is a curve present in the spine. When a curve is present, the spine rotates to keep everything aligned, and since the thoracic spine is what the ribs attach to, that rotation causes the ribs to create something that looks like a hump. If you've ever had a medical professional ask you to bend over so they can check the alignment of your spine, that is what they are looking for.

Normal Spine Test vs. One with Scoliosis

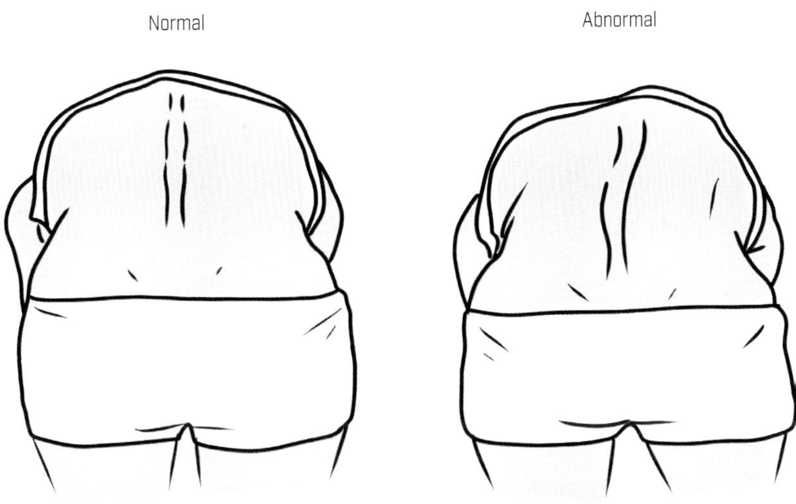

Ideally, scoliosis is tracked by a medical professional to make sure that the curve isn't becoming severe enough for other measures to be taken. It also helps to see a PT in person for a least a few visits to make sure you understand your specific curve and what it may be doing to your muscles and how you move.

If your curve is very minor and you have had it tracked in the past, one of the best things you can do is general strengthening. You can start by doing the lower back-strengthening exercises starting on page 106 and the mid back-strengthening exercises starting on page 120. While going through the exercises, make sure you feel the muscles on both sides of your body working equally hard. The stronger you get in the muscles that surround the spine, the more support your spine will have in the long term.

RHOMBOIDS AND THORACIC PARASPINALS

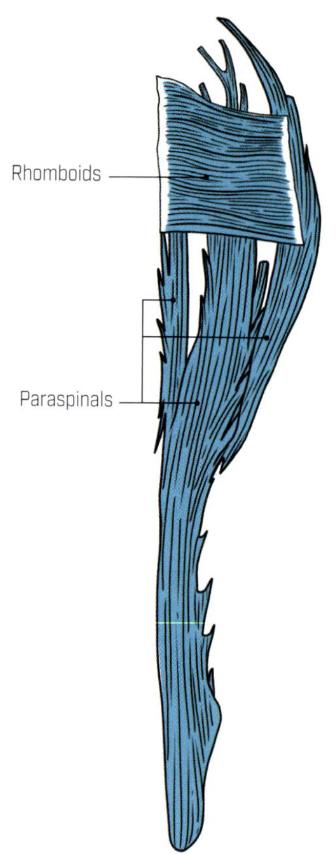

The two main muscles that can cause discomfort in the mid back are the rhomboids, which connect the inside of the shoulder blades to the spine, and the thoracic paraspinals, which run parallel to the thoracic spine.

These muscles can be incredibly stubborn and can be the main source of the stiffness you feel in your mid back. The best way to start to reduce the tightness in these muscles is by using a lacrosse ball to follow the self-massage techniques on pages 117 and 118. It is also important to do the thoracic mobilizations starting on page 119, because if your thoracic spine is stiff from spending so much time in an overly rounded position, these muscles will likely also feel stiff and tight.

Along with that, it is important to do the mid back– and shoulder-strengthening exercises found on pages 120-21 and 157-58, respectively. When you have discomfort and tightness in your mid back muscles, it may be because they are weaker than they should be. It could also be because they are overcompensating for weakness in the shoulder, especially the rotator cuff. So, strengthening both areas is the best way to ensure you are covering all of your bases.

RIB HYPERMOBILITY AND SUBLUXATIONS

Another diagnosis that can cause consistent tightness and discomfort in the mid back muscles is an unstable rib segment. Whether the rib is hypermobile (meaning that the ligaments that connect the rib to the spine are loose, causing the rib to move more than it should) or the rib subluxes (the rib actually moves out of its position), the body will respond by tightening these muscles to try to regain some stability.

I've had a lot of people refer to this as "slipping a rib," and it happens quite often in some populations. Doing a lot of activity or taking a blow or pressure to the rib cage itself can cause it.

If you have this diagnosis, taking a deep breath or coughing will likely cause pain. Since the ribs are basically a protective cage for your lungs, when there is a rib issue, any action of the lungs will also cause discomfort.

When this is the case, the thing you want to avoid is pressure over the ribs, including foam rolling. Foam rolling or using a lacrosse ball can exacerbate the reason everything is painful in the first place. You want to avoid pressure on the rib cage to allow those ligaments to heal. That is why it's important to determine whether the muscular discomfort you're feeling is coming from stiffness in your thoracic spine or something that is moving too much.

As your symptoms calm down, you can start to gently do the mid back mobilizations on page 119 and the mid back–strengthening exercises on page 120. Allowing your rib cage to slowly heal while also gently getting back the range of motion and building strength and stability through the region are the best ways to reduce this pain.

LATISSIMUS DORSI TIGHTNESS

The latissimus dorsi (lat) is the biggest muscle in the mid back, and when it is tight, it can create discomfort anywhere along the muscle. Most commonly, it is felt toward the outside of the body under the shoulder blade or up in the armpit where the lat attaches.

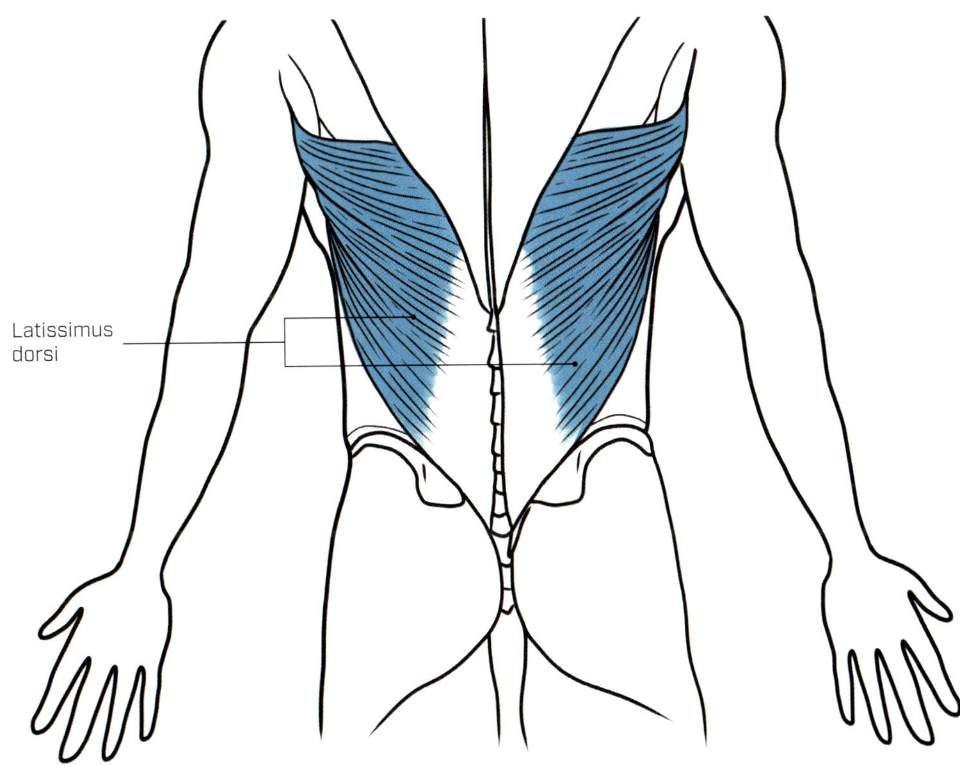

This muscle can become tight for the same reason that the mid back becomes tight, so it is a good idea to do the prayer stretch on page 119 and the mid back mobilizations found on pages 119 and 120. The lat tends to respond very well to stretching and mobilizations, especially if you do them multiple times a day.

The lat may also become tight if you spend very little time raising your arms above your head. If you have ever had major shoulder surgery or suffered from a case of frozen shoulder, you may have gone months without lifting that arm overhead. Since the lat moves the arm down and close to the body, if you aren't raising your arm up and away from your body, the lat is kept in a shortened position. So, along with focusing on the mobilizations and the stretch, make sure you are finding ways to get your arms away from your body throughout the day. This can be as simple as sitting up and reaching your hands up toward the ceiling as far as you can go.

REFERRED PAIN FROM THE NECK

If what you're feeling in your mid back is more of a tingling, burning, or numbness, there is a good chance that it is coming from somewhere in the neck. The most common culprit is a muscle called the levator scapulae. Since this muscle attaches to the top inside corner of the shoulder blade, when it is tight, it can cause a tingling pain along the inside edge of the shoulder blade. You can read about what to do for levator scapulae tightness on page 124.

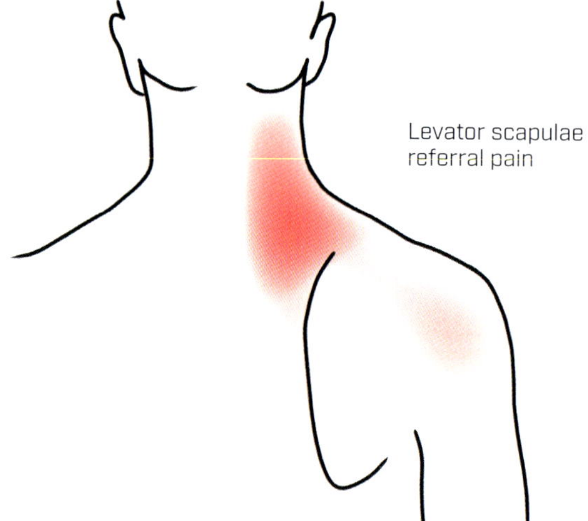

If you feel an occasional tingling but mostly a big pulling sensation when pointing your head downward, then that is also coming from your neck. This sensation can be caused by tightness in a few different areas of the neck, but by following the neck mobilizations, stretches, and exercises starting on page 130, you can reduce that tightness in your mid back.

When dealing with anything in the mid back, it is always a good idea to also address your neck *and* shoulders since they are so closely tied to this area.

SELF-MASSAGE TECHNIQUES & MOBILITY, FLEXIBILITY, AND STRENGTHENING MOVEMENTS FOR THE MID BACK

SELF-MASSAGE

LACROSSE BALL

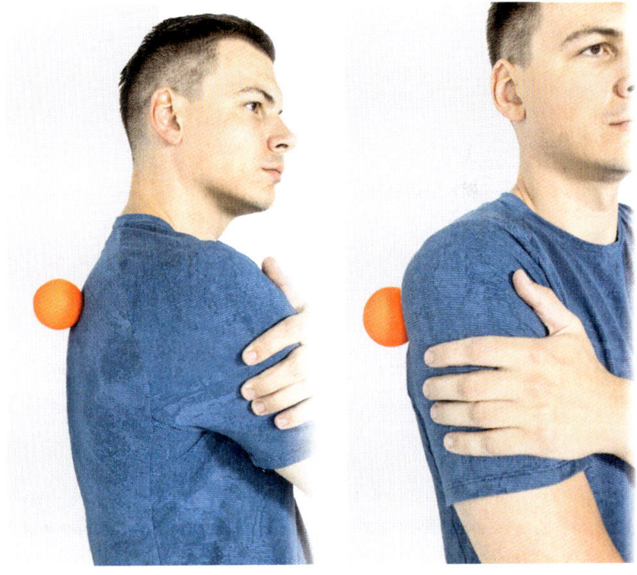

To get to specific muscles in the mid back, the best tool to use is a lacrosse ball. While leaning with your back against a wall, roll the ball between your back and the wall, trying to target the rhomboids and thoracic paraspinals that were discussed on page 114. Maneuver your body around, finding tight and tender muscles. Using gentle pressure, you can make small movements to create a massage in the area. You can also just lean into a tight spot with gentle pressure and take deep breaths. Don't spend longer than three to five minutes on an area, and make sure that the pressure you're using is gentle enough that you feel better when you're done. You can repeat this as needed.

FOAM ROLLER

To massage the muscles more broadly, you can use a foam roller while lying on the floor. Cross your arms in front of you and use your feet to rock your body forward and backward along the roller. Repeat for three to five minutes, and then use the foam roller to do a gentle mobilization.

Move your butt down so it's sitting on the floor. Position the foam roller in a stiff spot of your mid back and lean back into the roller until you feel gentle pressure. Hold for a second or two and then come back to where you started. Feel free to try different parts of your mid back, making sure that you are going gently enough that you don't increase your soreness.

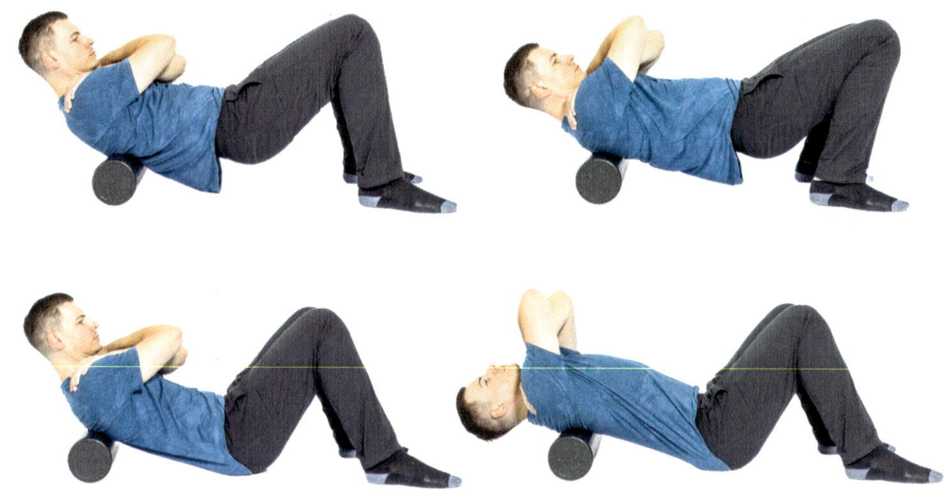

STRETCHES

FOAM ROLLER STRETCH

Standing facing a wall, place the foam roller on the wall at about the height of your chin. Place the sides of your hands on the roller with your shoulders rounded forward slightly. Roll your hands up the wall, and as the foam roller gets higher than your head, bring your chest in toward the wall. You should feel a stretch in your armpits and a slight pressure in your mid back. Once you feel that stretch, hold for two to five seconds and repeat ten times. You can do this as needed.

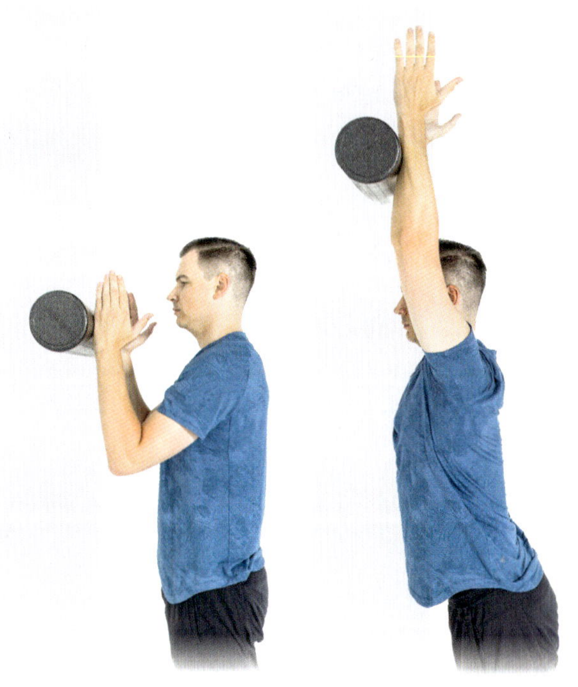

PRAYER STRETCH

Sitting in a chair at a desk or table, place the backs of your arms on the desk in front of you and keep your palms together. Keep your chest up tall as you move your butt backward and bend forward at the waist. Once you feel a gentle stretch in the armpit area, hold for fifteen to twenty seconds and repeat three times. You can do this as needed.

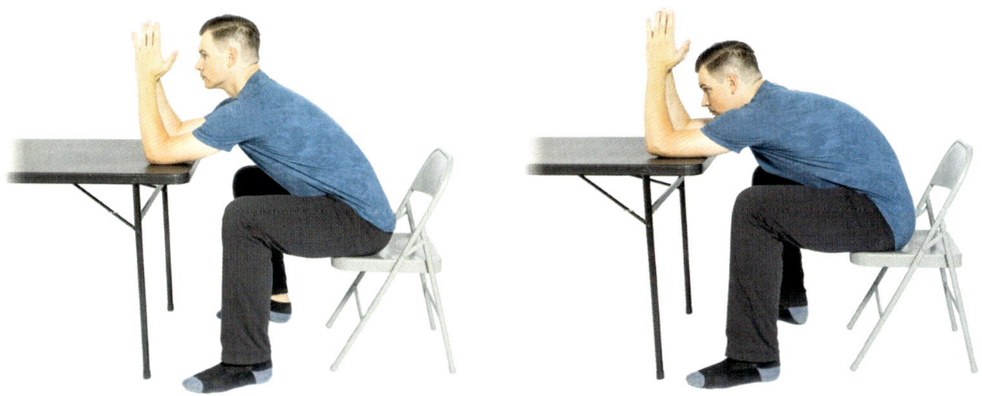

MOBILIZATIONS

THORACIC/MID BACK FLEXION AND EXTENSION

Sit up tall in a chair with your back not touching anything and cross your arms in front of you. Start by trying to bend forward using only your mid back. Keeping your lower back from moving, round your mid back forward as far as you can and hold for about a second. Then try to move as far as you can in the opposite direction by thinking about pointing your chest toward the sky. Once again, you should be making this movement without moving your lower back at all. Hold that position for about a second and repeat ten times in each direction. Feel free to repeat this movement as needed.

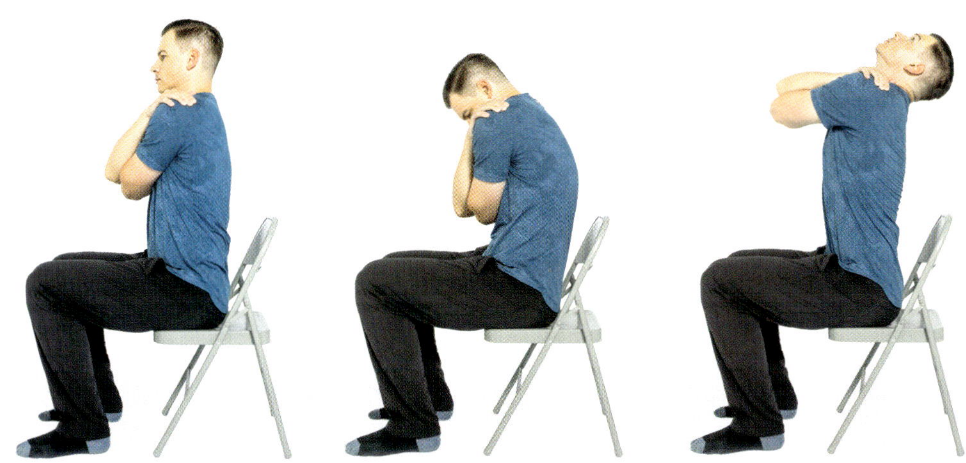

OPEN BOOKS

Lie on your side with your arms straight out in front of you. Without allowing your hips to move, slowly move your top arm across your body, creating a gentle twist. Stop when you feel a gentle stretch or pressure in either your chest or your mid back, and repeat ten times on each side. Feel free to repeat this movement as needed.

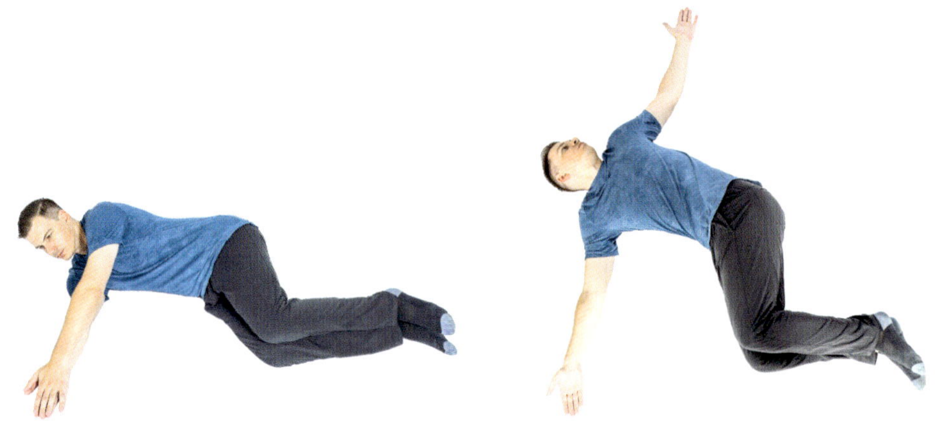

STRENGTHENING EXERCISES

For all of these exercises, secure a resistance band out in front of you at about belly button height. Choose a band strength that feels challenging but still allows you to go through a full range of motion. You will likely be able to use a stronger band for the rows than for the other two exercises. For each exercise, you want to keep your shoulders in a down-and-back position. This will force the muscles of your mid back to work and not allow the muscles of your neck to overcompensate. If at any point you feel the neck muscles taking over, step away and reset your shoulders in that down-and-back position. For all of these exercises, repeat for three sets of ten and do them daily.

The easiest way to do this is by tying a small knot in the middle of a resistance band. Then slide that small knot through an open door, just above the middle hinge. When you close the door, the band will be secured at about the right height for everyone.

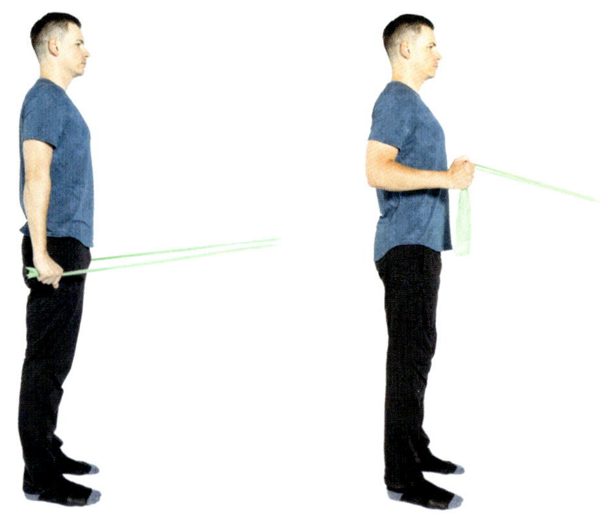

STANDING Y'S

Hold onto the ends of the band with your arms straight and your palms facing the ground. While keeping your shoulders down, raise your hands up over your head, creating a "Y." If you are keeping your shoulders low, you should feel this exercise working the muscles in the backs of the shoulders all the way down to below the shoulder blades.

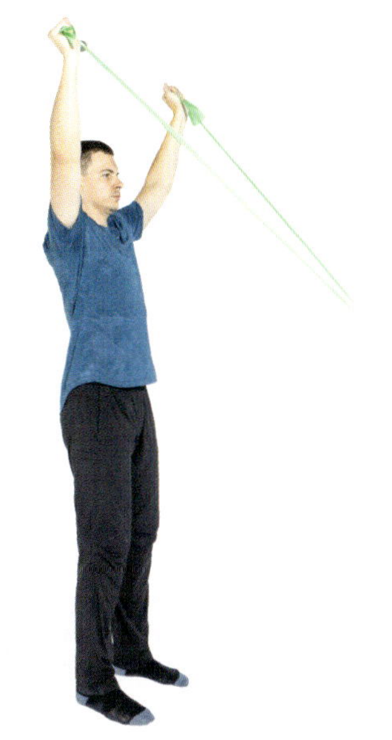

ROWS

Hold onto the ends of the band with your arms straight out in front of you and your palms facing each other. Think about bringing your elbows straight backward while imagining that you are trying to squeeze a pencil between your shoulder blades. Once you feel like your elbows can't go back any farther, return to where you started.

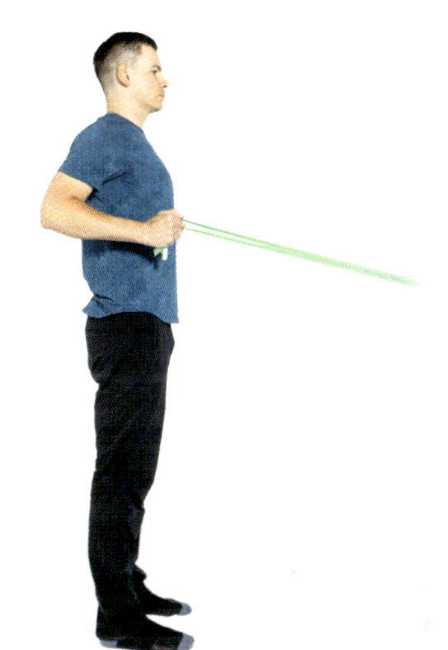

SHOULDER EXTENSIONS

Hold onto the ends of the band with your arms straight out in front of you and your palms facing the ground. Keep the shoulders low and arms straight as you bring your hands down by the sides of your hips. You should feel this working the muscles of the back. Once you get your hands to the level of your hips, return to where you started.

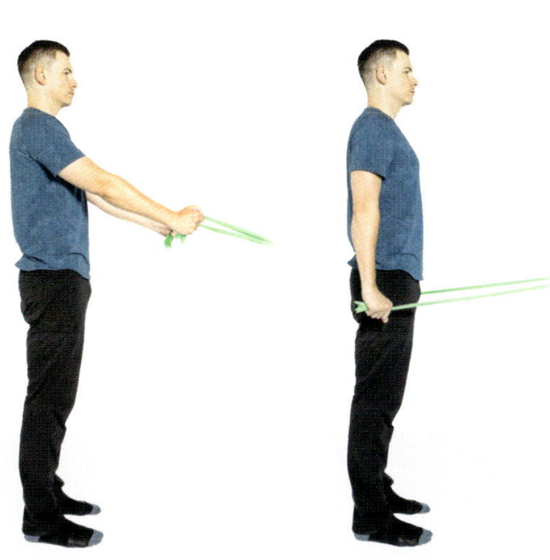

SECTION 5

THE NECK, THE HEAD, AND THE JAW

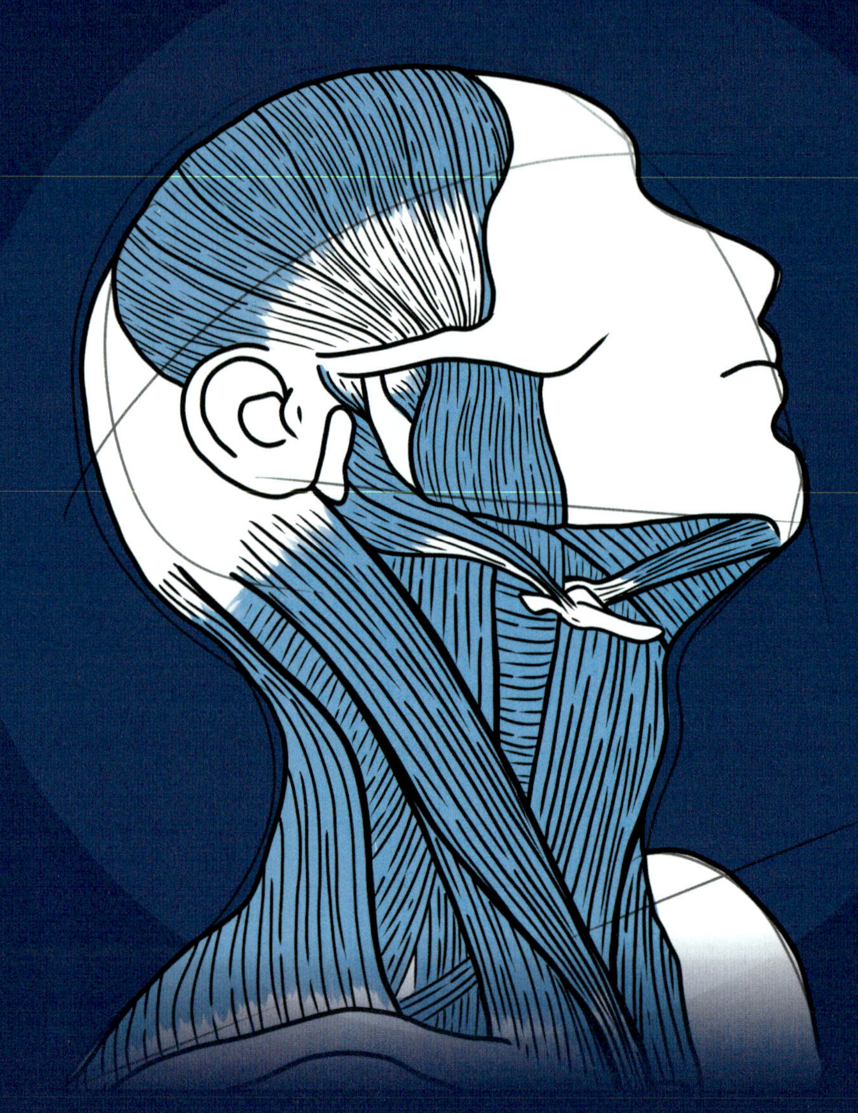

The lumbar spine makes up the lower back, the thoracic spine makes up the mid back, and the cervical spine makes up the neck. The cervical spine is made up of seven vertebrae stacked on top of one another with vertebral discs between them, just like the other sections of the spine. The top two cervical vertebrae look different from the other five because they are responsible for supporting the skull. Along with that, there are nerves, arteries, veins, and muscles that form the rest of the neck and create an intricate system in which a lot of little aches and pains can pop up.

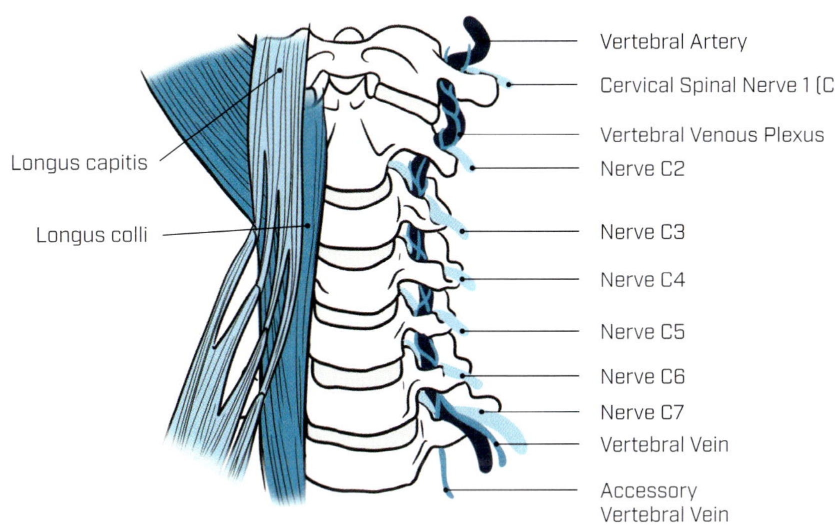

Neck pain has become increasingly common as people spend almost all of their waking hours sitting and staring at a screen. Even if you have a perfect ergonomic set-up, the neck has trouble standing up to the hours of operating a phone and a computer all day, every day. It's no secret that prolonged sitting and awkward head positions while looking at a screen can lead to neck pain, but so can strenuous activity and even stress.

If you mostly have neck pain following activities like exercising or doing household chores, then make sure you also read the section on the shoulder, specifically the rotator cuff, beginning on page 141. Neck pain following activity is heavily related to the muscles of the neck overcompensating for weakness in the rotator cuff. Especially if you feel like your neck pain hasn't responded to stretches and exercises that involve the neck, the shoulder may be your culprit.

If you find that your neck pain is mostly due to stress in your life, try this:

Take a deep breath in through your nose and exhale very slowly through your mouth. As you exhale, try to allow your shoulders to completely relax as you allow them to lower down to the floor. If you felt like your shoulders dropped significantly, then you are likely holding a lot of tension through the muscles of your neck, and repeating a breathing exercise like this every twenty to thirty minutes can be extremely helpful.

THE UPPER TRAPEZIUS [TRAP], LEVATOR SCAPULAE [SCAP], AND FIRST RIB

I'm lumping these three structures together because it is rare to have an issue with one and not the other two. So, when addressing discomfort associated with one, you will have a lot more success if you don't ignore the others.

The upper trapezius muscle (trap) is the largest muscle in the neck. Since it is so big and expansive, it gets a lot of the blame for any tightness in the neck. However, in my experience, the more stubborn muscle is the slightly smaller levator scapulae (levator scap). This thin muscle runs from the top inside corner of the shoulder blade all the way up into the neck and can be the main source of tension that you feel anywhere in that area. Along with these two muscles, I have also listed the first rib, which sits a lot higher in the body than most people realize. When these two muscles are tight and pull your shoulders up toward your ears, the first rib can also feel stiff in this lifted position and cause discomfort.

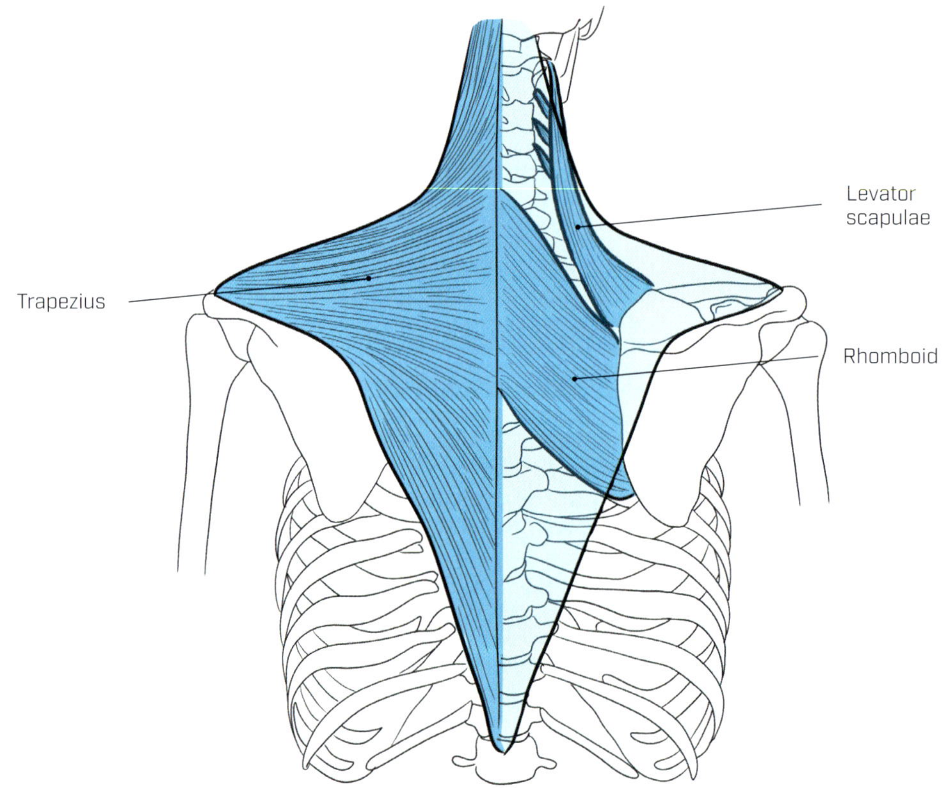

When you have an issue in any of these three areas, you mostly just feel a general stiffness or tightness that never seems to go away. The discomfort can present itself anywhere throughout these muscles or in the first rib.

As mentioned above, when there is tightness in these areas, it is important to work on the strength of the rotator cuff in the shoulder. In the clinic, about 95 percent of people with tightness in this area also seem to have weakness in the rotator cuff. So, along with reading through this section, be sure to read the section on the rotator cuff starting on page 141.

Also mentioned previously, this is a common area to hold stress. So doing the breathing exercise on page 132 along with simply being aware of where you are holding your stress can be extremely helpful. If you sit and work at a desk, it is also important to make sure you are working with your arms in a supported and relaxed position. The easiest way to do that is by allowing your forearms to be fully supported on the desk. If your forearms aren't supported, the only things holding up the weight of your arms are these two muscles, and keeping them active all day long can lead to a lot of tightness and discomfort. Just making the change to supporting the forearms and feeling like you can work and type with your shoulders totally relaxed is all some people need to make a complete reduction in their symptoms.

Finally, you can do the stretches listed on pages 135 and 136 throughout the day to make sure you are keeping this area as loose and mobile as possible. If you follow through on all of this, you should notice a significant difference in your symptoms in just two to three weeks.

Even if your issue is with some of the smaller muscles in the neck not mentioned here, like the scalenes or the paraspinals, the small movements that I give for those muscles are the same movements I have suggested here. There is a lot of overlap in the suggested movements and exercises for the neck, so getting into every single small muscle would lead to a lot of redundancy. Since the traps and levator scaps are the major muscles in this area, if you take care of them, the other muscles will likely follow suit.

JOINT PAIN

Joint pain in the neck most commonly presents as pressure, pinching, or tightness in the back of the neck, and it primarily occurs when looking up. This is most commonly associated with arthritis and stenosis in the vertebrae of the neck, but it can also occur in people who spend a lot of time in a forward head posture. When you have irritation in the joints of the neck, anything that compresses the back of the neck will increase your symptoms. If there is enough compression in the area, it can even start to compress nerves and cause a pain down into the arm. This nerve pain would also increase as you look up and compress the joints in the back of your neck.

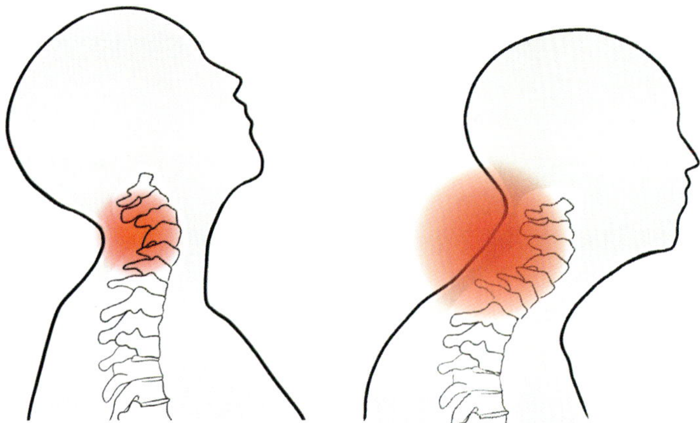

If you experience pain when getting into either of those two positions, the easiest way to reduce your symptoms is by doing the chin tuck mobilization on page 134. This movement creates space in the joints of the neck, reducing compression and therefore reducing symptoms. You can do the chin tuck standing, sitting, or lying on your back, and it's a good idea to do it multiple times throughout the day.

Along with using the chin tuck to reduce symptoms, you can also use it as an exercise (see page 137) to build up the strength of the front of your neck. When you experience pain in the back of the neck, one of the best things you can do for the long-term health of the neck is to build strength in the front. This is an overlooked muscle group, and the weaker the muscles are in this area, the more likely you are to fall into a forward head posture and increase discomfort.

These two movements will help the most, but it is also a good idea to strengthen the shoulders with the exercises found on pages 157 and 158. As with other issues in the neck, the weaker the shoulders are, the more strain is placed on the muscles of the neck.

INSTABILITY

If you have instability in the joints of the neck, you may feel like your head becomes extremely heavy by the end of the day. Sometimes it can feel so heavy that you need to support it with your hands or lie down because you don't have the strength to support your head anymore. You may also feel chronic tightness in all of the muscles of the neck since they are all working overtime to help stabilize the cervical spine. Especially if you know that you are hypermobile or "double jointed" in other areas of the body, this is likely what is going on.

If you are unstable or hypermobile, there is unfortunately no stretch or mobilization that will truly help to reduce your symptoms. You may have already figured this out for yourself. Since your symptoms are coming from trying to support the neck and head, the best thing to do is strengthen the muscles of the neck. The neck exercises found on pages137 and 138 may be very difficult at first, but the more you do them and the easier they become, the more stable your head and neck will feel, and hopefully the symptoms will subside.

When doing these exercises, it's important to feel like the muscles are working, but you do not want to increase symptoms. You also don't want to do so much that you feel so fatigued that you can't hold up your head afterward. Once you find a sweet spot of working the muscles without too much fatigue or an increase in symptoms, do the exercises daily for at least two to four weeks.

DISC PAIN

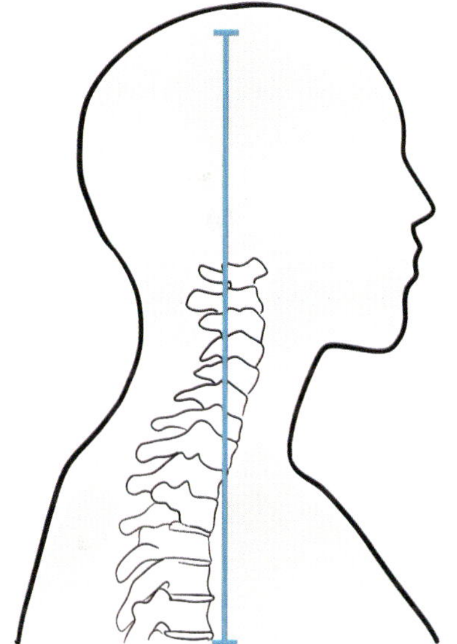

When people think of a herniated disc, they mostly think of the discs in the lower back. However, you have discs between the vertebrae throughout your entire spine. While injuring one in the low back is far more common, you can also injure the discs in your cervical spine. (For more information on the anatomy and the discs in the spine, refer to "The Lower Back" starting on page 95.)

The most common way to injure a disc in the cervical spine is by lifting something heavy or pulling or pushing something with great force. You can also slowly injure the back wall of a disc over time with poor mechanics of the spine.

The two hallmark signs of a disc injury in the neck are an increase in pain while looking down and an increase in pain with an increase in pressure, such as sneezing or coughing. The pain most often starts where the disc injury is, but since the disc is so close to the nerves that run down the arm, it can also cause shooting pain along the track of that nerve. So, if you sneeze or cough and feel immediate nerve pain anywhere in your arm, there's a good chance that this is what you're dealing with.

Since looking down increases strain to the disc and increases pain, it's a good idea to stay away from the neck stretches. It's also a good idea to take a break from lifting, pulling, or pushing heavier objects for at least a couple of weeks. As much as possible, you want to keep your head in a neutral position to reduce stress on the disc and allow it to heal. Whether sitting or standing, you want to maintain this neutral position. It is also helpful to do the symptom-reducing technique found on page 132.

As your symptoms decrease, you can start to do the chin tuck mobilization found on page 134. Start very small and be very gentle. The more you do, the more you can push into it, but you don't want to rush the process. It should always feel comfortable and should never increase your symptoms. Once those mobilizations become easy, you can add the neck exercises on pages 137 and 138. Finally, it's a good idea to do the shoulder exercises starting on page 120 as well to make sure your shoulders can properly support your neck.

STERNOCLEIDOMASTOID (SCM) PAIN

The sternocleidomastoid is a mouthful of a muscle that is more affectionately known as the SCM. The SCM is one of the more literally named muscles in the body because it runs from the sternum (sterno) and clavicle (cleido) all the way up to the mastoid process (mastoid), which is very close to your ear. This muscle will most commonly cause tightness and discomfort in the front of the neck, but it can also cause pain around the ear where it attaches.

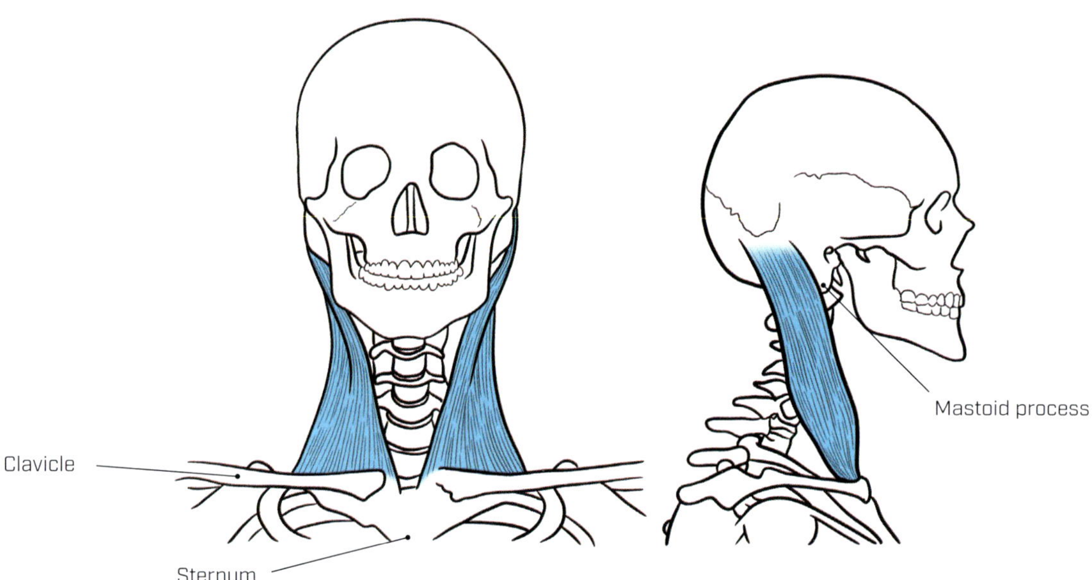

In my experience, when the SCM is upset, it is mostly because it is overcompensating for other muscles. So, along with doing the SCM stretch on page 136, make sure you are also doing the neck and shoulder exercises found in this book. As you reduce tension in the SCM with the stretch and provide more support by strengthening the other muscles, you should notice a significant difference in just a few weeks.

THE HEAD AND THE JAW

When it comes to the head and the jaw, there are two main areas that I work on in physical therapy: headaches caused by tension in the muscles of the neck and jaw pain caused by dysfunction in the temporomandibular joint. Outside of these two areas, there isn't much that falls under the treatment of physical therapy.

If you are experiencing headaches that don't align with what I describe in this book, please seek out other medical guidance. Similarly, if you are experiencing a jaw pain that isn't helped by what I've written here, be sure to see a dentist or other oral care practitioner for guidance.

TENSION HEADACHES / REFERRED MUSCLE PAIN HEADACHES

The most common form of headache that is directly caused by tightness in the neck is referred to as a tension headache. These headaches occur when there is so much tightness in the area right below the base of the skull that the pressure causes pain in the head, typically either in the back of the head or in the forehead. While this is the most common presentation, there are a lot of other headaches that are commonly caused by other areas in the neck.

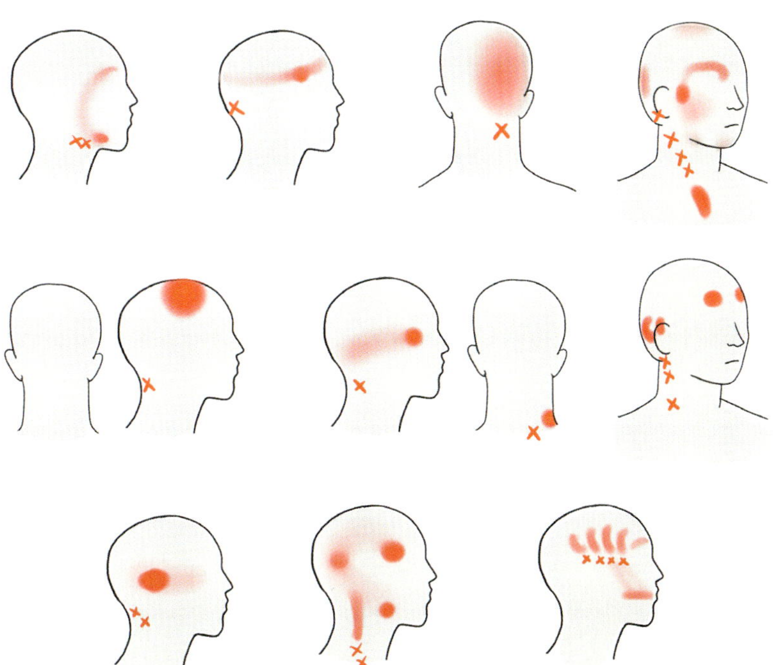

Especially if you feel tightness in the muscles of the neck already, the pain that is presenting in the head is almost certainly influenced by those muscles. Since there can be a lot of overlap in terms of what muscles are causing what pain, it's a good idea to read through the entire neck section to see what you align with. And since there are referral headaches that can be caused by the muscles in the jaw, it's also a good idea to do the self-massage techniques found on pages 133 and 134.

As symptoms start to decrease, it is a good idea to do neck- and shoulder-strengthening exercises to ensure that the muscles are strong enough to support the head and reduce the likelihood that they get tight enough to cause this pain.

TEMPOROMANDIBULAR JOINT (TMJ) PAIN

The temporomandibular joint (TMJ) is a fairly complicated joint that can be painful if any of the components aren't doing their job. The joint itself is where the top of the mandible meets the temporal bone, and a disc between the two bones is what allows the jaw to move and gives you the ability to yawn, speak, and eat. The main muscles in the area that can lead to pain are the temporalis, masseter, and pterygoids.

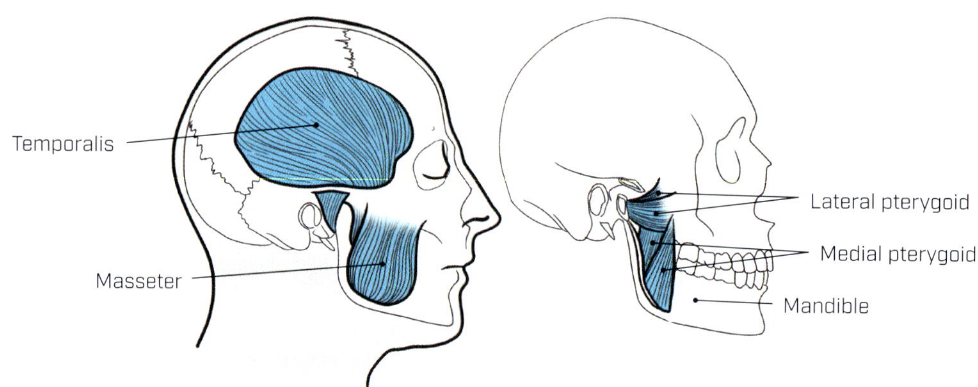

When this area is in pain, you may feel constant tightness and discomfort right around the joint, and you may even feel a clicking or popping sensation when opening and closing your mouth. This pain can be influenced by teeth grinding, stress, and even the position of the neck.

If you know that you are a teeth grinder, especially at night, then you should see a dentist and ask about a night guard. Especially if you feel like most of your jaw discomfort occurs first thing in the morning, the grinding taking place at night may well be the main cause of your pain.

If you find that your jaw pain increases with stress, then you can try the stress relief technique on page 132. Stress can not only lead to more teeth grinding but also create tension in the muscles that surround the jaw, which increases pain.

Finally, if you find that your jaw pain increases with movement like eating or talking, then the best place to start is with the self-massage techniques found on pages 133 and 134. If self-massage over the muscles makes a significant difference in your symptoms, then you can do it daily.

It's also a good idea to strengthen the muscles of the neck to make sure that the head is supported. One thing that will always stick with me from PT school is one of my professors saying, "If you have no idea what to do for someone's jaw, just treat their neck." That's because the muscles and position of the neck have so much influence over how the jaw moves and operates. If you focus on nothing more than the neck, you can still make a huge difference in the symptoms felt in the jaw. Therefore, doing the strengthening and flexibility movements for the neck that are outlined in this book is a great way to reduce the pain felt in the jaw.

If you feel like you get to the point where the pain has really gone down and your jaw feels better overall, but you still feel a click every time you open your mouth to a certain point, you can try the following exercise.

Open your mouth to the point right before you know you will feel the click. Then place your fist underneath your chin and press your chin into it. You want to feel like you are trying to open your mouth wider, but the fist is blocking it. Hold for two to three seconds. After repeating this five times, see if you can open your mouth slightly more without feeling a click. The goal of the exercise is to build strength and control in the muscles of the jaw. The more you do, the wider you can open your mouth before the click takes place. The goal is to repeat this exercise on a daily basis until you can open your mouth with no clicking in your jaw.

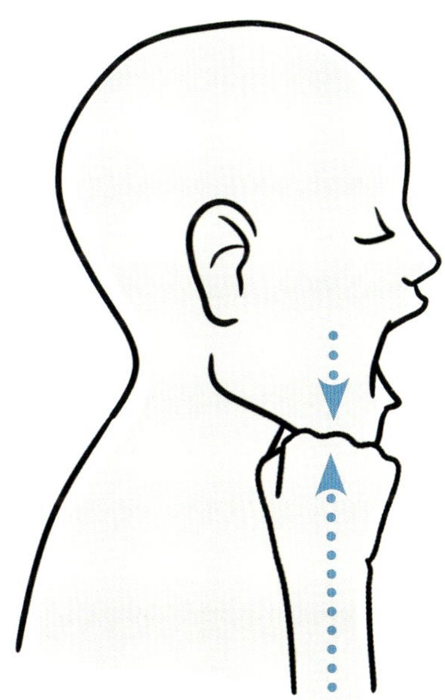

SELF-MASSAGE TECHNIQUES & MOBILITY, FLEXIBILITY, AND STRENGTHENING MOVEMENTS FOR THE NECK, HEAD, AND JAW

Before we dive into these movements, I would like to share a technique for overall symptom relief. Since so much of the pain felt in the neck, head, and jaw can be tied to stress, this is my favorite way to get that musculature to let go and calm down. It is not only my favorite way to reduce stress-related tightness but also useful to do before the other techniques I'm about to go over.

Find a place to lie on your back with your feet elevated. The best place to do this is often on the floor near a couch or a chair. Put your legs up, roll up a towel, and place it behind your neck. From there, take deep breaths in through your nose and out through your mouth. With each exhale, you want to feel your head and neck relax. When you have your head and neck relaxed, focus on other body parts. Once you feel like you have gotten your full body to relax, you should feel a significant difference in stress-related symptoms.

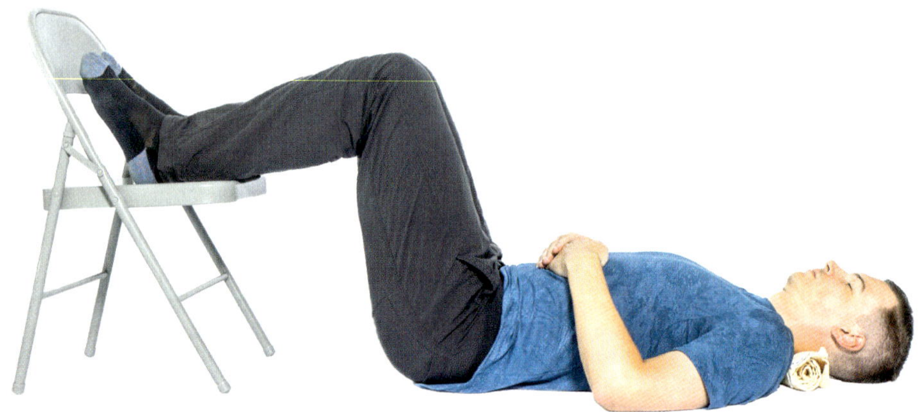

SELF-MASSAGE

TEMPORALIS (JAW) MASSAGE

Your temporalis runs from the temple area of your forehead and attaches to the jaw. Lying on your back, take your first two fingers and place them on your temple. With firm pressure, find tight and tender spots in that muscle and massage with small circles. Continue to gently massage the area for two to five minutes.

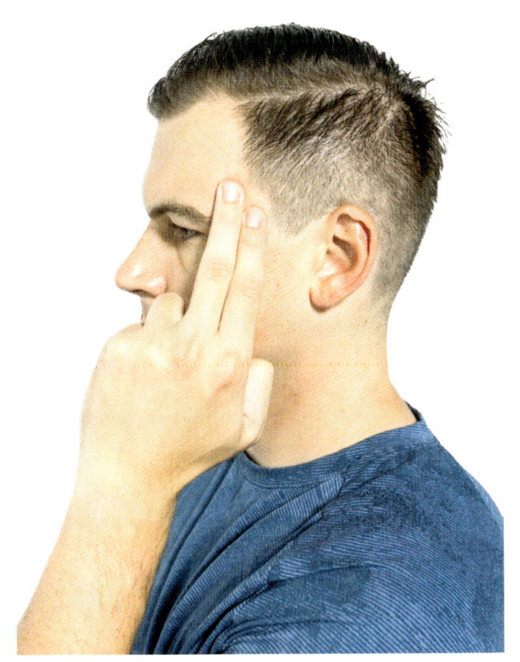

MASSETER (JAW) MASSAGE

The masseter is the biggest muscle in the jaw and the main muscle that allows you to chew and grind. To locate it, all you have to do is clench your teeth with your fingers on your cheek. The muscle you feel controlling the jaw and popping into your hand is the masseter. To massage it, place your first two fingers over the muscle with your thumb pressing into the mandible for stability. With firm pressure and your jaw fully relaxed, massage the muscle with small circles. Find tight and tender spots, and continue to gently massage the area for two to five minutes.

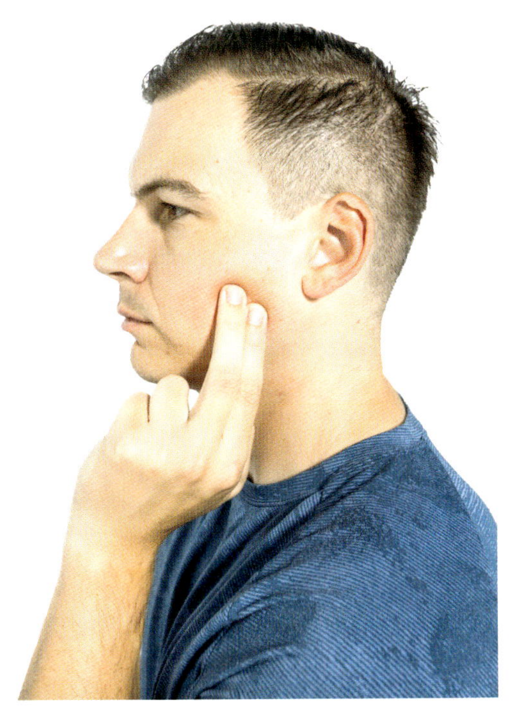

PTERYGOIDS (JAW) MASSAGE

The pterygoids are a pair of small muscles that you can massage from the inside of your mouth. This is the muscle group that attaches to the disc in the TMJ, so tightness here can influence the clicking in the jaw that you may sometimes feel. To massage it, run your index finger along your bottom molars until you reach the end. From there, bring your finger toward your cheek and raise it up toward your top molars. This is where you should feel a small, rope-like muscle. This muscle may be extremely tender, so start with very gentle pressure and run your index finger up and down the length of the muscle for one to three minutes. The muscle should loosen up very quickly, and when it does, you may notice an immediate reduction in clicking in the jaw.

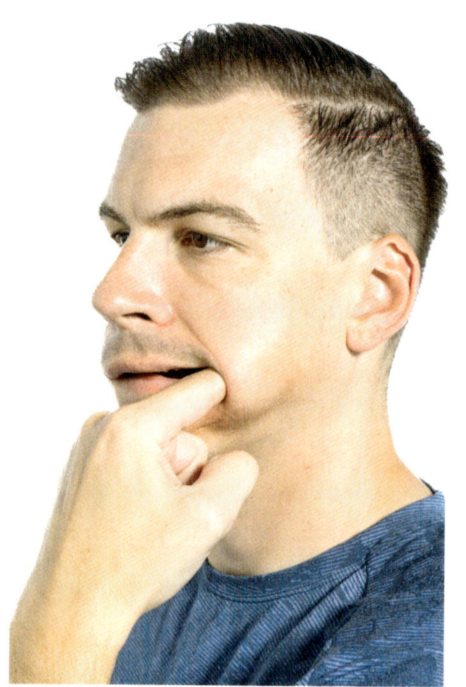

MOBILITY

CHIN TUCKS (NECK/TENSION HEADACHES)

Chin tucks can be used to mobilize the joints of the cervical spine since the chin tuck position creates more space in the joints. Lying on your back, lower your chin as if you were trying to give yourself a double chin and focus on flattening the back of your neck against the ground. Once you feel a gentle stretch in the back of your neck, hold for one to two seconds and repeat for two sets of ten.

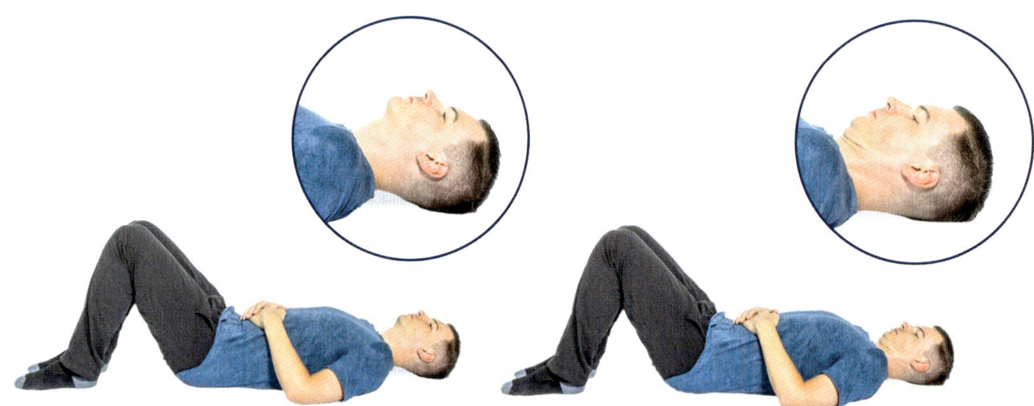

FIRST RIB MOBILIZATIONS (NECK/UPPER TRAP AREA)

Sitting up tall, take a bath towel and twirl it up on itself to make it tight. Place the towel where your shoulder meets your neck on the side you want to work. Pull the towel down with as much force as you can apply and stabilize it with the other hand. Maintaining that pressure, tilt your head in the opposite direction until you feel a gentle stretch (you will not be able to go very far). Hold the gentle stretch for one to two seconds and repeat for two sets of ten.

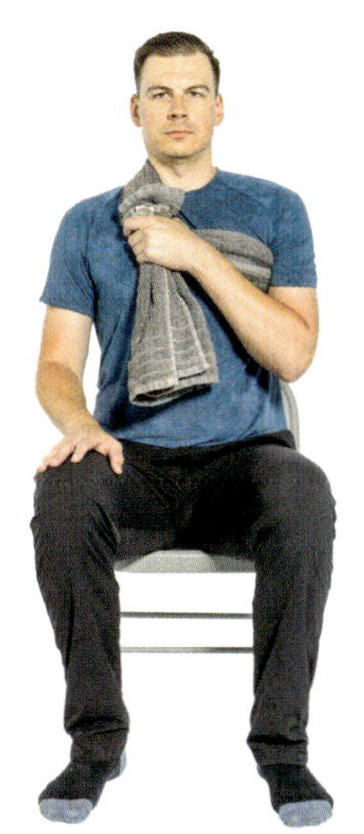

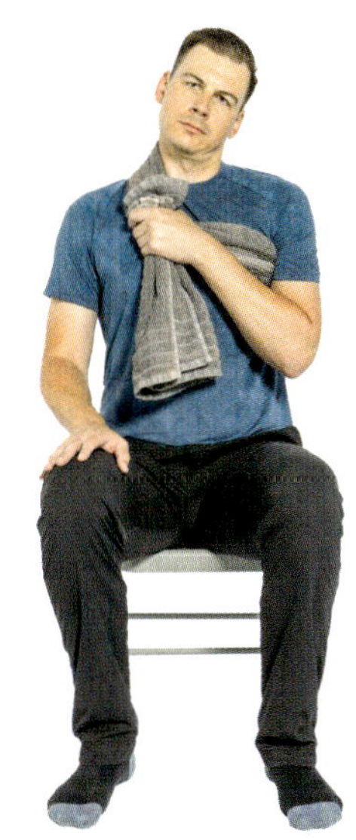

STRETCHES

UPPER TRAP STRETCH (NECK)

Sitting up tall, sit on the palm of your hand on the side you intend to work. From there, just tilt your head in the opposite direction until you feel a gentle stretch. Hold for fifteen to twenty seconds and repeat three times.

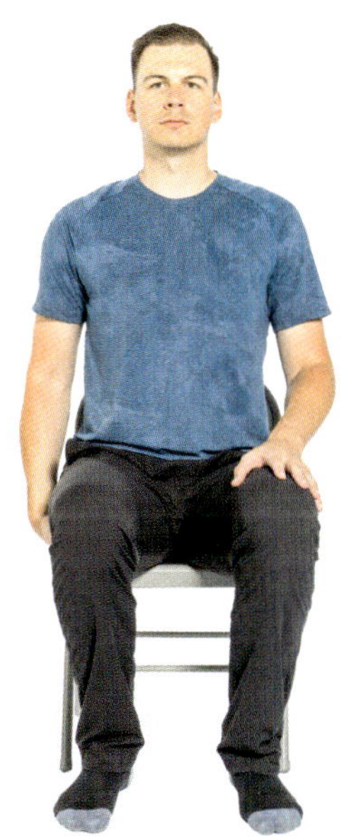

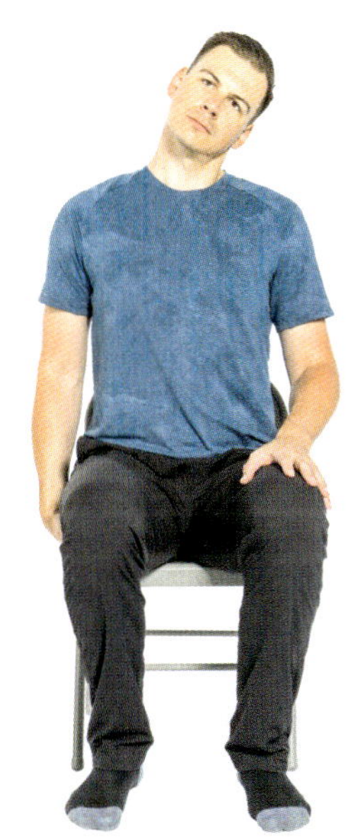

LEVATOR SCAP STRETCH (NECK)

Sitting up tall, sit on the palm of your hand on the side you intend to stretch. From there, bring your nose down and across your body toward your opposite armpit. Once you feel a small stretch, keep your chin tucked and move your chin toward the middle of your chest until you feel an even bigger stretch. Hold for fifteen to twenty seconds and repeat three times.

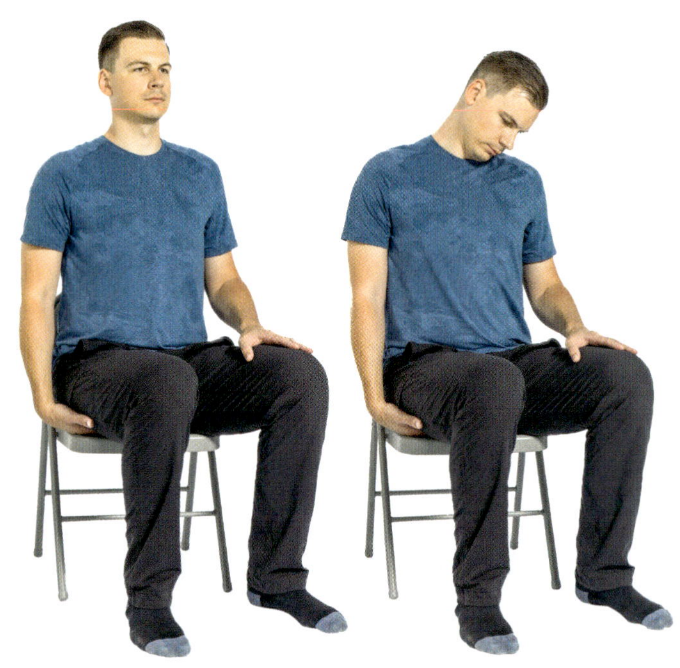

SCM STRETCH (NECK)

Sitting up tall, place your hand on the collarbone of the side you intend to stretch. Point your chin up and away from that collarbone until you feel a gentle stretch in the front of your neck. Hold for fifteen to twenty seconds and repeat three times.

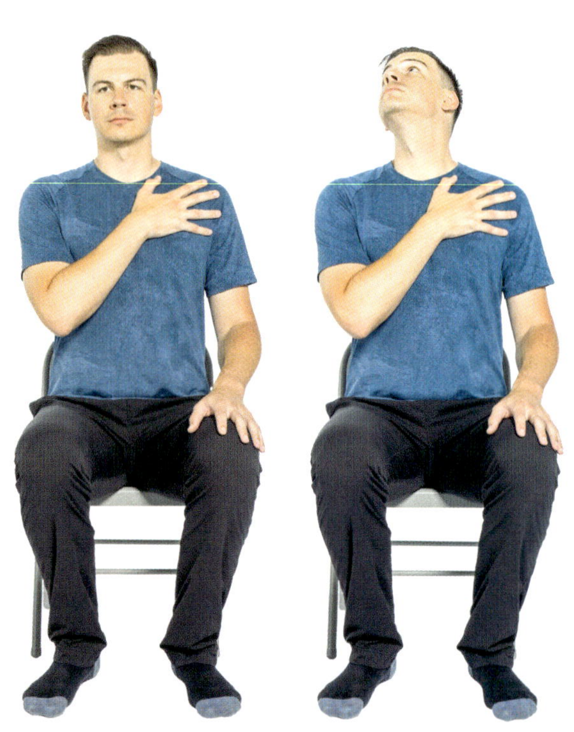

STRENGTHENING EXERCISES

CHIN TUCK CURLS (NECK)

Lying on your back with your knees bent, tuck your chin in as you did for the chin tuck mobilization. Continue to move the chin in that direction until the back of your head begins to come up off the floor. If you are maintaining the correct position, you should not be able to move your head very far. Once you have your head about an inch or two off the ground, try to hold for ten to fifteen seconds. You should really feel the muscles in the front of your neck working, and this may feel very difficult at first. Repeat for three sets of three. As the exercise gets easier over time, try to increase the hold to twenty to thirty seconds.

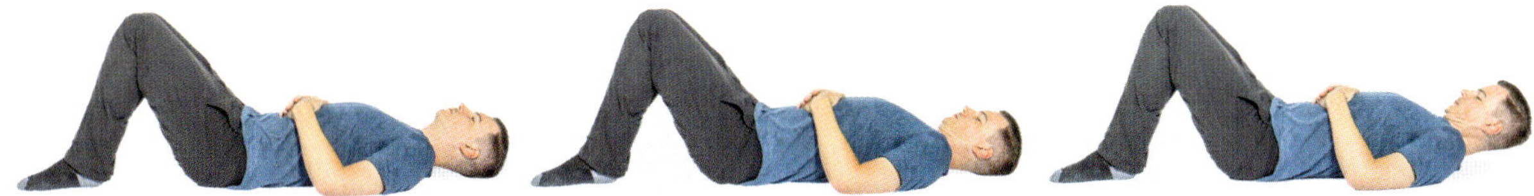

CHIN TUCK WITH ROTATION (NECK)

Lying on your back with your knees bent, tuck your chin in as you did for the chin tuck mobilization. Keep your chin tucked as you turn your head to one side as far as you can. Keep the chin tucked as you come all the way back to where you started, then relax. Tuck your chin again and repeat the movement to the other side. Do this ten times.

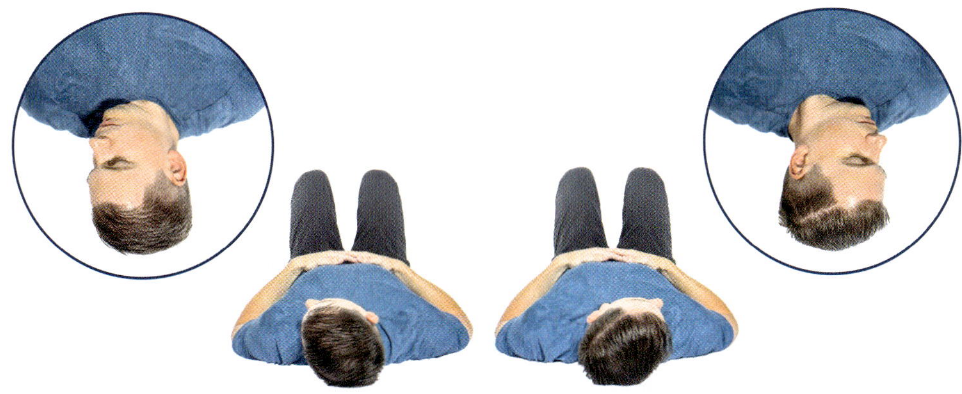

NECK SIDE PLANKS (NECK)

Lying on your side, simply try to keep your head in a neutral position while keeping it as stable as possible. You should feel like you are using the muscles on the side of your neck that is facing the ceiling. Hold this position for fifteen to twenty seconds and repeat three times on each side.

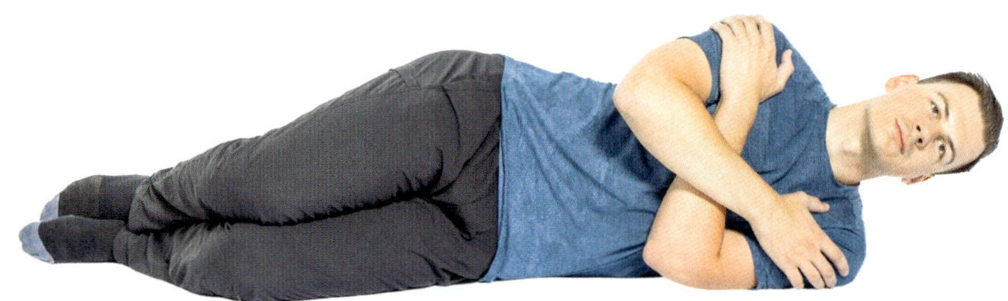

SECTION 6

THE SHOULDER

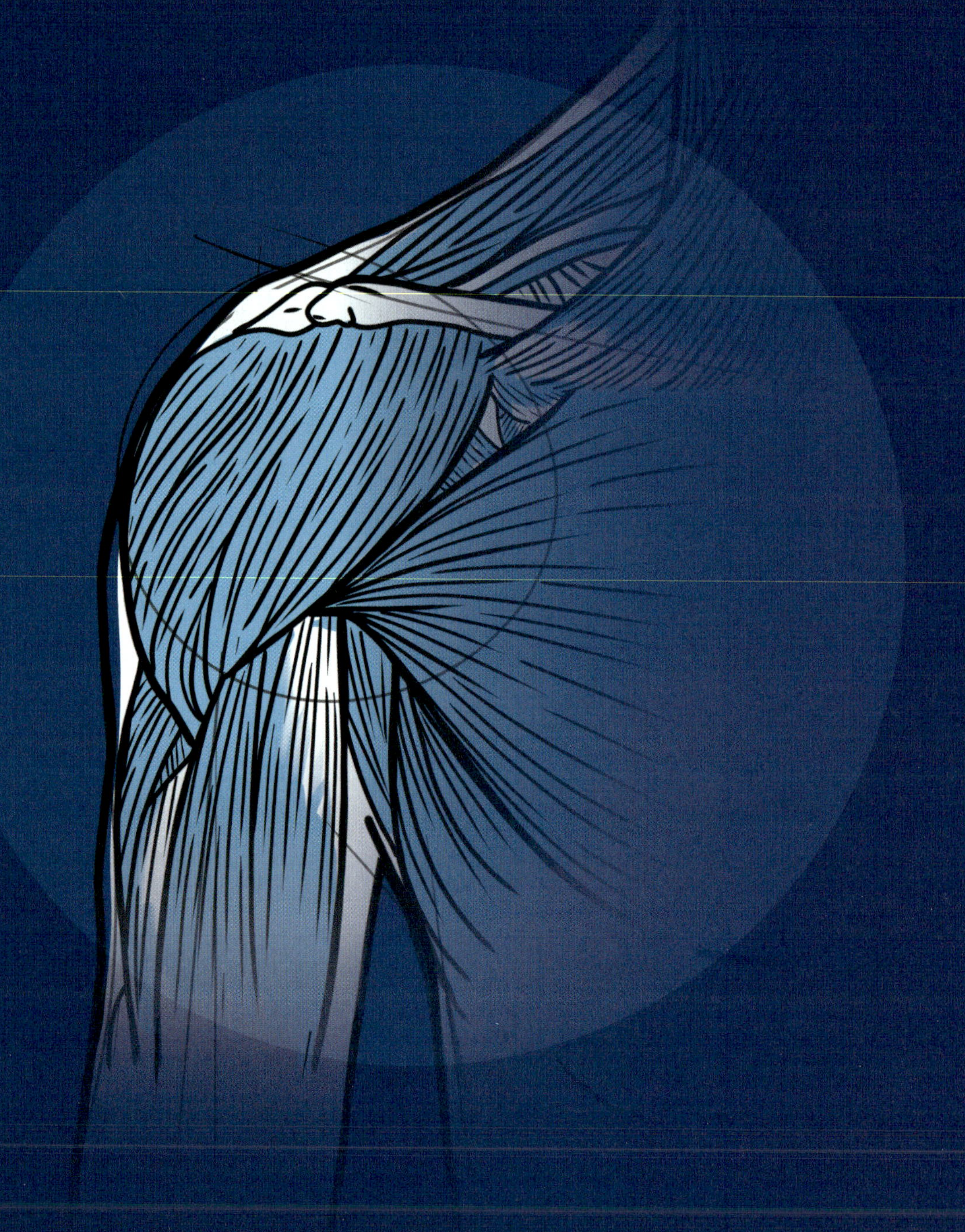

Before I started my career in physical therapy, my lifelong dream was to be a professional baseball player. I'd played the game my whole life, but my career was limited by my shoulder health. I always felt like there was more that I could do for my shoulder, so I dedicated a large part of my professional life to taking down the main obstacle that held me back. Shoulder injuries are extremely personal to me. While I try to give every patient and every diagnosis the same level of thought and energy, the shoulder cases still hit a little differently.

Arguably the most complicated joint in the human body, the shoulder has by far the most range of motion of any joint, and it takes a lot of muscles to facilitate that range of motion. In my experience, the best way to address issues in the shoulder is to focus on the main source of control and stability: the rotator cuff. When there is discomfort or pain anywhere in the shoulder, it's hard to find a better place to start than the rotator cuff.

ROTATOR CUFF WEAKNESS

The rotator cuff is a group of four muscles. The subscapularis is the only one that lies on the inside of the shoulder blade, while the other three—the supraspinatus, infraspinatus, and teres minor—lie on the back of the shoulder blade. All four muscles attach around the head of the humerus to create one cohesive structure that is meant to provide stability to the shoulder joint while the shoulder moves, lifts, and reaches. If the rotator cuff isn't up to the task, then the surrounding muscles overcompensate to try to create the stability that the shoulder is lacking. This overcompensation leads to pain and tightness in the other muscles of the shoulder. Almost all pain and tightness anywhere in the shoulder or neck can be tied to weakness in the rotator cuff.

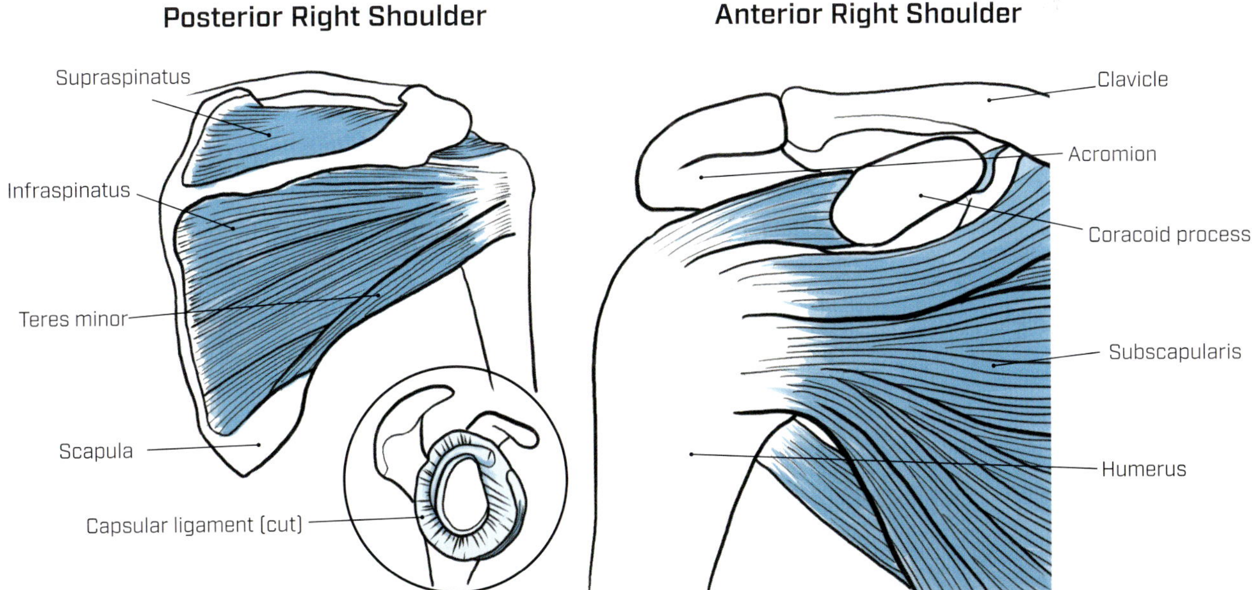

If you want to see if you have an issue with the strength of your rotator cuff, find a partner and stand facing them with your elbow bent to 90 degrees and your hand in a fist. Holding your elbow steady against your torso, have your partner try to move your fist away from your body while you resist with everything you have. If your subscapularis is healthy and strong, your partner should not be able to move your fist.

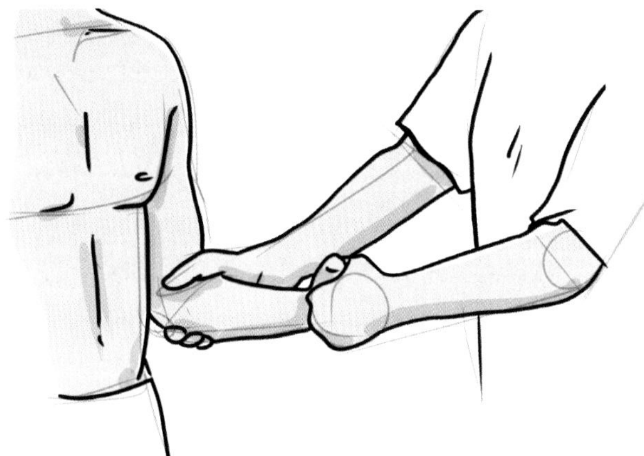

For the next test, keep your elbow braced against your torso and bent to 90 degrees, and move your fist away from your body. Have your partner try to move your fist back to the midline of your body as you resist. If your rotator cuff is strong and healthy, your partner should not be able to move your fist at all. But if your partner can move your fist, especially if they can move it with ease, weakness is likely contributing to your symptoms.

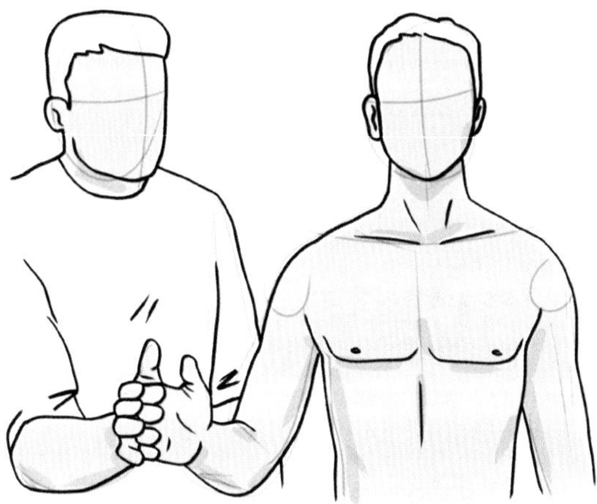

The best first step is to reduce tension in the rotator cuff muscles on the back of the shoulder blade by following the instructions in the "Self-Massage" section on page 154. Take just three to five minutes to roll out the muscles of the rotator cuff as instructed, and have your partner retest your ability to prevent them from moving your fist. If it greatly improves, that means your rotator cuff has the ability to be strong and active; it just needs a little help to unlock its potential. An immediate increase in strength also means that it is a good idea to roll out the shoulder in this way before doing the rotator cuff exercises on pages 157 and 158. For the most part, the rotator cuff is weak because the muscles are tight from overuse, and a tight muscle is a weak muscle. By taking away tension from the muscles, you can increase your ability to contract and use them.

When I have a patient with shoulder pain, one of the first things I look at is how easily I can move their fist as described. For the most part, they show weakness in the external rotators (trying to keep the fist from being pushed inward toward the body). After I massage the external rotators on the back of the shoulder blade for five to ten minutes (the same muscles in the "Self-Massage" section on page 154), they see an immediate increase in strength. The look of shock on their faces never gets old, and I often tell them that it's the only magic trick I know. It's the simplest example of how much easier it can be to use muscles once they are relaxed and not stuck in a tight and uncomfortable state. And it is how I prove that rolling out with a lacrosse ball should always be done before the exercises.

Most people who come in to see me with neck or shoulder pain on one side have this kind of rotator cuff tightness. After three to four weeks of rolling out the shoulder and doing the banded rotator cuff exercises on pages 157 and 158 three to four times a week, they start to notice a massive improvement in their pain. This is the building block of all of my shoulder evaluations. It is an easy way to start to get all of the symptoms to slightly decrease, because ultimately, if the rotator cuff is dysfunctional, then nothing in this region can truly get better.

As you'll see while reading through the rest of this section, most diagnoses in the shoulder tie back to the strength and control of the rotator cuff. Maybe if I had known that when I was fourteen years old, I would not be writing this book, because I would be too busy making millions of dollars pitching in the major leagues.

LABRUM INJURY

If the rotator cuff is the source of muscular stability in the shoulder, the labrum is the source of structural stability. The labrum is fibrocartilage that encapsulates the head of the humerus in a similar way to the rotator cuff. It is the "socket" that forms a suction cup for the "ball" of the "ball and socket" joint of the shoulder. The health of the labrum is closely tied to the health of the rotator cuff because if one of them is compromised, it places more stress on the other one. And because they are so closely tied together, if you injure one, you have also likely injured the other. My baseball career ended with a tear in both my labrum and my rotator cuff, but through understanding the joint and dedicating myself to my own rehab, I was able to avoid surgery, and I have helped plenty of others do the same.

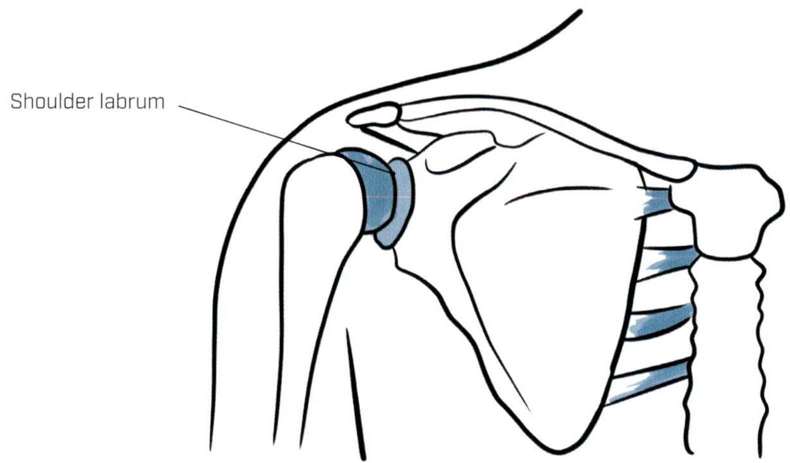

A labrum injury most commonly presents as an inability to stabilize the shoulder. This can be due to a tear, general laxity or hypermobility, or following a dislocation. When the labrum loses its ability to stabilize the shoulder, more stress is placed on the rotator cuff, and this can be one of the main causes of an overworked rotator cuff.

If you have significant pain in your shoulder when moving it in any direction, you feel a "clunk" in your shoulder when moving it at a certain angle, or you feel like your shoulder is always about to dislocate, see an orthopedic or sports MD, as it might mean you have a tear and need imaging. People can recover from small tears in the labrum with exercise, but if the tear is too big or the labrum itself has become too lax, you may need surgical intervention.

The goal of exercise is to build enough strength and control in the rotator cuff to allow the labrum to heal. In my case, I know that as long as I continue to do my rotator cuff exercises a couple of times per week, my shoulder feels just fine, and I get to stay off the surgical table.

ADHESIVE CAPSULITIS (FROZEN SHOULDER)

Frozen shoulder, or adhesive capsulitis, is the opposite of the labrum being too lax or loose. It develops when inflammation takes over the shoulder and tightens the shoulder capsule to the point where range of motion is limited in all directions. This can happen after a fall or even after bumping your shoulder on something, but it is most prevalent in middle-aged to older adults, especially if a comorbidity such as diabetes is present. Once the inflammatory process starts, little can be done to slow it down or improve the shoulder before it is ready.

Frozen shoulder commonly progresses through three stages:

- **The "freezing" stage:** Pain increases, and you notice that your shoulder is getting tighter and you are losing range of motion.
- **The "frozen" stage:** Pain decreases, but the shoulder is still very stiff and hard to move.
- **The "thawing" stage:** Pain continues to go down, and you notice that your range of motion is finally coming back.

Frustratingly, these stages can last for six months to over a year. The mobility and flexibility exercises on pages 155 and 156 will help you maintain as much range of motion as possible, but it's important not to "fight" against the shoulder or push yourself into significant pain. If you irritate the shoulder, you can increase the inflammation and make your symptoms worse.

As you reach the "thawing" stage, you can start to push the mobility and flexibility exercises slightly harder and also begin doing the strengthening exercises. However, it is important to focus on getting your full strength and range of motion back to avoid future injuries.

THE FRONT OF THE SHOULDER

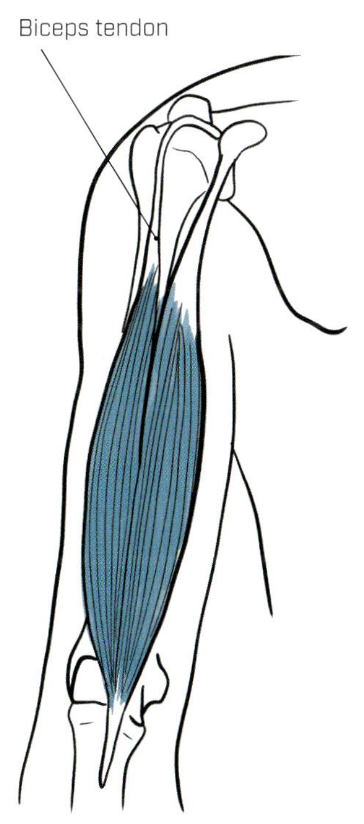

BICEPS TENDON PAIN

One of the most common causes of pain in the front of the shoulder is irritation in the tendon of the long head of the biceps muscle. To see if this is the source of your pain, simply press your thumb deep into the front of your shoulder and move it back and forth. If you feel a tight, rope-like structure under your thumb that is irritated and painful when you press into it, the biceps tendon is likely the cause of your symptoms.

Pain and irritation in the biceps tendon commonly results from overworking the biceps. You may also notice that you have a lot of tightness in the biceps muscle itself. Address it by doing a stretch for the biceps (see page 156) and eccentric biceps curls with a light weight that doesn't increase your symptoms (see page 171). As you do these two things to address the biceps, you should notice a significant improvement in your shoulder symptoms.

However, it is also possible that you have a labrum issue. The biceps tendon attaches to the labrum, and if the labrum is compromised, the biceps tendon can get extremely irritated. If you have pain in the biceps tendon but no real tightness in the biceps muscle, then you should approach this as a labrum issue. Go back to page 143 and follow the instructions there.

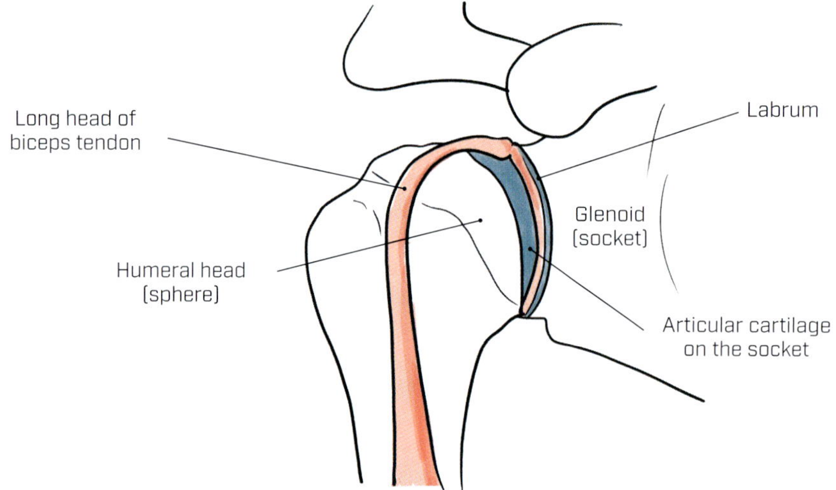

AC SPRAIN

The acromioclavicular (AC) joint is where the acromion process of the scapula meets the clavicle (collarbone). The ligaments of the AC joint are meant to hold it steady, but if you sustain an injury in a fall or are creating repeated stress to this area via overuse, then it can become painful. Most people feel the pain right over the joint itself, and pain can increase with movement of the shoulder, especially overhead or in pushing movements like push-ups and bench presses.

AC Joint

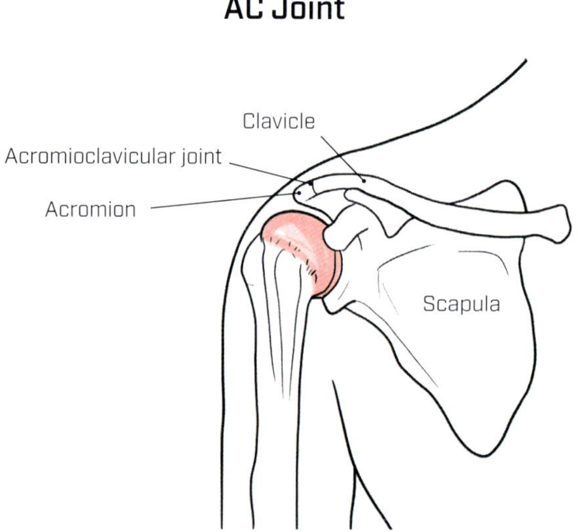

Since this is a sprain, it's important to protect the area like with any other sprain. First, do not do any movements that provoke symptoms. As the pain subsides, you can start to do the shoulder mobility movements found on page 155, as long as you don't irritate symptoms. As your range of motion improves, you should also focus on the strength of the rotator cuff, especially if the sprain resulted from overuse.

SHOULDER IMPINGEMENT SYNDROME

If you're feeling pain in the subacromial space, just below the acromion process, especially when moving the arm, then you are likely dealing with a shoulder impingement. This occurs when structures beneath the acromion process get pinched because of inflammation, swelling, or inefficient movement of the shoulder.

Subacromial Space and the Structures Within It

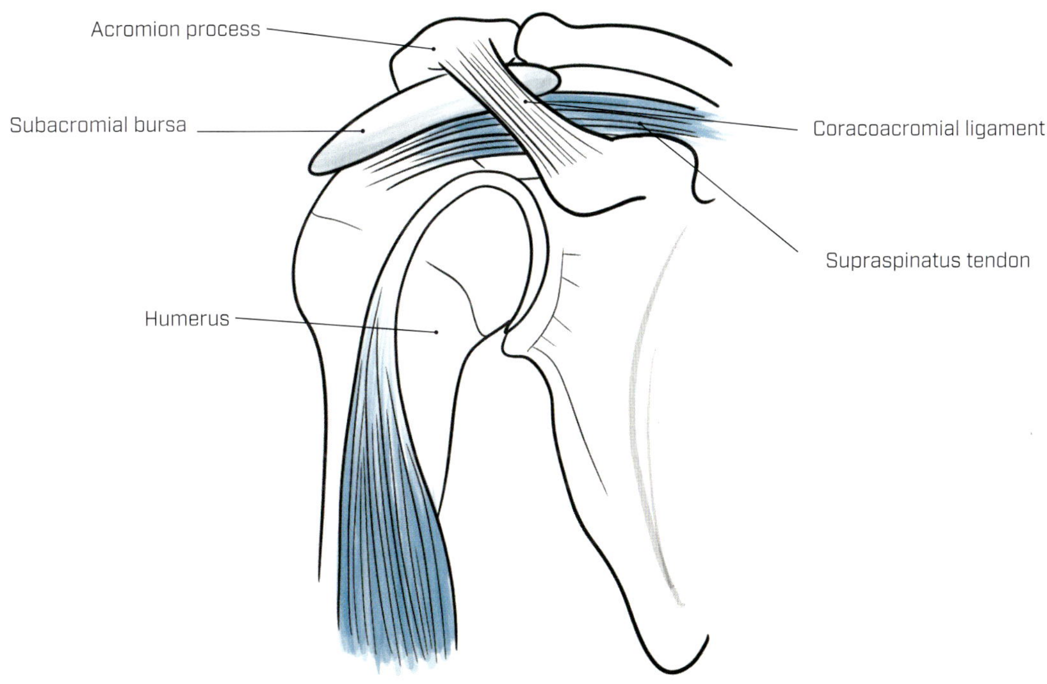

The hallmark of shoulder impingement is known as a "painful arc," or when movement of the shoulder is painful only when lifting it to around shoulder height, because that creates pressure in the subacromial space. Lifting the arm below or above shoulder height is not as painful because more space is created and the structures are no longer being impinged upon.

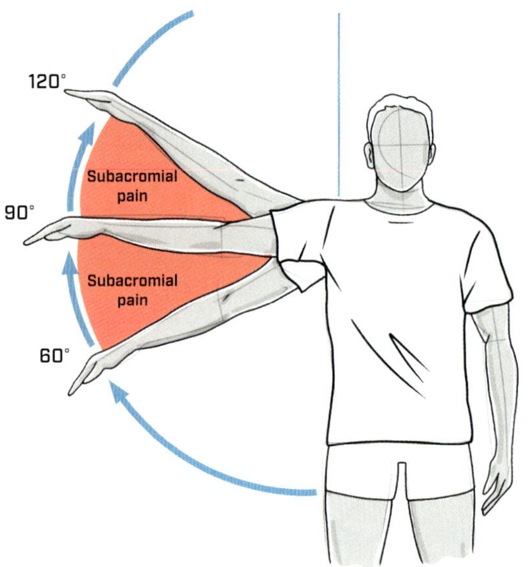

Positive test result: Shoulder pain between 60° and 120° indicates subacromial or rotator cuff disorder

To start dealing with this pain, try the wall slides found on page 155. Using the wall for a little extra stability will allow you to raise your arm through the "painful arc" with hopefully minimal to no pain. Ultimately, the impingement is likely happening because of weakness or a lack of control in the rotator cuff, so doing the rotator cuff exercises found on pages 157 and 158 will also address symptoms. As you improve your strength and work on mobility, normal and pain-free movement should return.

SC SPRAIN AND COSTOCHONDRITIS

Two different diagnoses irritated by similar movements, a sprain at the sternoclavicular (SC) joint occurs where the sternum meets the clavicle (collarbone), and costochondritis pain occurs mainly where the sternum meets the ribs.

This pain can be caused by compression in these joints from excessive pushing movements like push-ups or bench presses or by spending a lot of time lying on your side with your shoulders rounded forward. In the case of costochondritis, the pain can be so

SC Joint and Where the Ribs Meet the Sternum

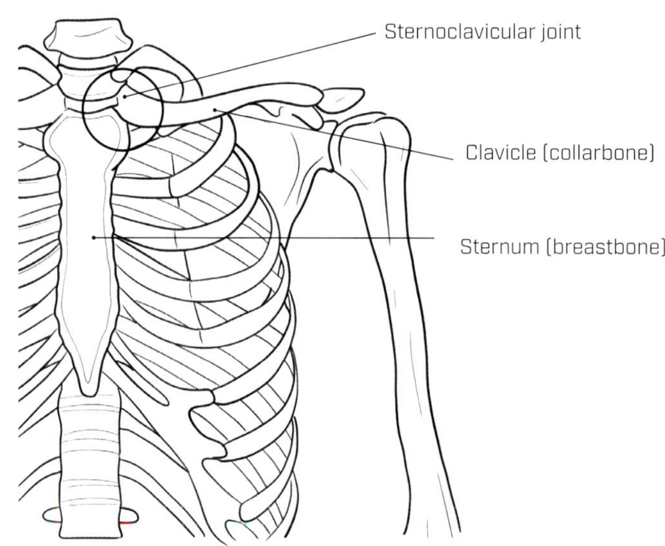

intense that it is sometimes mistaken for a heart attack. The main way to differentiate this pain from a heart attack is to press directly over the area where the ribs meet the sternum. If pressing on that area re-creates your symptoms, then costochondritis is the likely source. Also, since the collarbone and ribs move when you take a deep breath, that can also re-create pain.

Just to be safe, it's always nice to have a refresher on what the American Heart Association lists as the six signs of a heart attack:

1. Chest pain or discomfort
2. Pain or discomfort in the jaw, neck, or back
3. Pain or discomfort in the arms or shoulders
4. Shortness of breath
5. Feeling very tired, lightheaded, or faint
6. Nausea or vomiting

They suggest calling 911 if you or someone with you is experiencing one or more of these symptoms.

The best way to start to reduce symptoms is to protect the area by avoiding any movements that increase your symptoms. Stop lying on your side and instead opt to lie on your back. If you notice that your symptoms worsen after movements like push-ups and bench presses, then reduce either the number of repetitions you are doing or the weight you are using for a few weeks. As your symptoms decrease, you can start doing the pec stretch on page 156 and the shoulder mobility exercises on page 155 as long as they don't stir up any pain. As symptoms continue to improve, it's also a good idea to improve the strength of the rotator cuff with the exercises on pages 157 and 158.

PECTORAL MUSCLE TIGHTNESS

You have two pectoral muscles in your chest: the pectoralis major and the pectoralis minor. The pectoralis major is the muscle that you think of when you think of someone's "pecs." This is the larger and more external muscle that really grows when you dedicate yourself to exercises like push-ups and bench presses. This muscle can become tight and irritated, but the problem child of this two-sibling family is almost always the pectoralis minor.

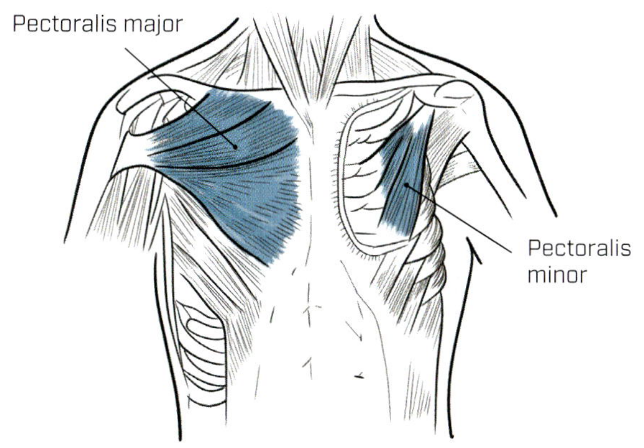

This muscle lies underneath its major counterpart and can create pain in the front of the chest or shoulder. Overdoing exercises can be the culprit, but so can spending a lot of time with your shoulders in a rounded position—working at a desk, scrolling on your phone, or sleeping on your side curled up into a ball.

The best way to start to address tightness in this area is by doing the pectoralis stretches on page 156. And if you notice that you are spending prolonged periods of time with your shoulders in a rounded position, it is a good idea to find ways to limit that. This can be as simple as taking time throughout the day to sit up straight and pull your shoulders into a down-and-back position. And much like costochondritis, if you notice that your symptoms always worsen after movements like push-ups or bench presses, reduce either the number of repetitions you are doing or the weight you are using for a few weeks.

It is also a good idea to work on the strength of the muscles of the rotator cuff (see pages 157 and 158) and those in the mid back (see pages 120 and 121). The stronger these muscle groups are, the easier and more natural it will be to prevent your shoulders from rounding forward.

THORACIC OUTLET SYNDROME

When I have a patient in the clinic who is experiencing numbness or a tingling sensation traveling down into the arm, I first look at the possibility of it being caused by one of the joints or discs in the cervical spine.

If the impingement isn't taking place there, then it is likely happening in the space where the torso meets the shoulder, known as the thoracic outlet.

The thoracic outlet is where major nerves, arteries, and veins exit the neck and torso and enter the shoulder to travel down the arm. If something in this outlet is impinging upon any of those structures, it can cause numbness, tingling, and sometimes pain that travels down the arm and often all the way down into the fingers.

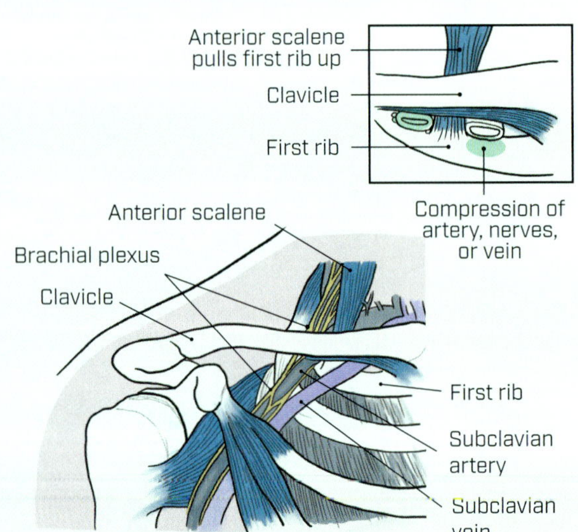

When thoracic outlet syndrome is present, there are three likely culprits: the first rib, a muscle called the scalene, or the pectoralis minor. The first rib and the neck musculature are addressed on pages 124 and 125, and the pectoralis minor is addressed on pages 149 and 150. To start to address this syndrome, follow the advice listed for both areas. Numbness should lessen over the course of a few weeks.

If it doesn't, it's a good idea to see a professional in person sooner rather than later. There are a lot of possible causes of numbness in the arm, and it's best to find out the root cause as soon as possible.

THE SIDE OF THE SHOULDER

When I see someone who is experiencing pain on the outside of the shoulder, the most likely culprit is the rotator cuff (see page 141). The most common cause of pain in that area is referral pain coming from the rotator cuff.

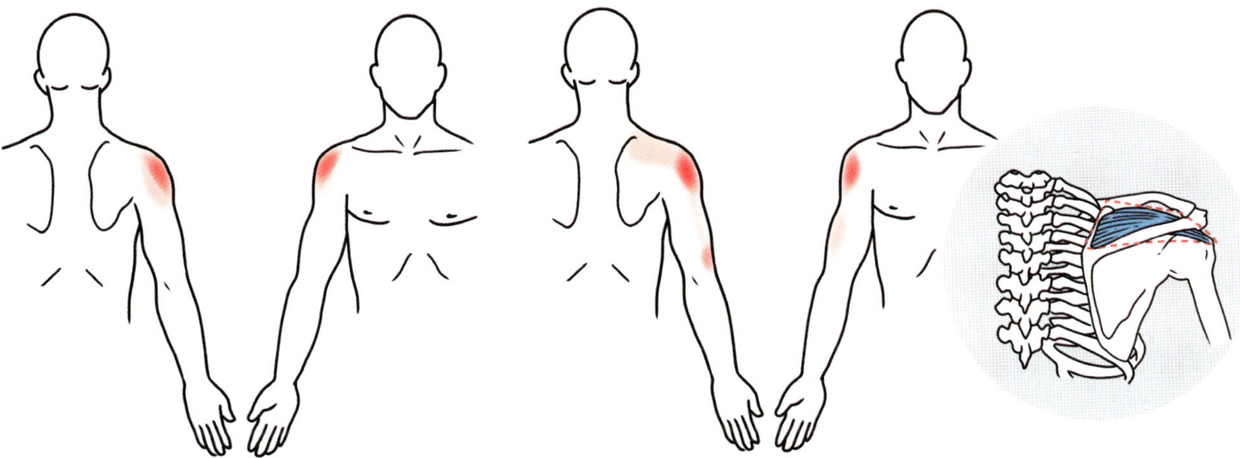

If, instead of pain in the side of the shoulder, you are feeling a deep pain that seems to wrap around the outside of your shoulder, it may be a referral pain coming from the labrum (see page 143). This pain is often described as a dull ache coming from deep within the shoulder.

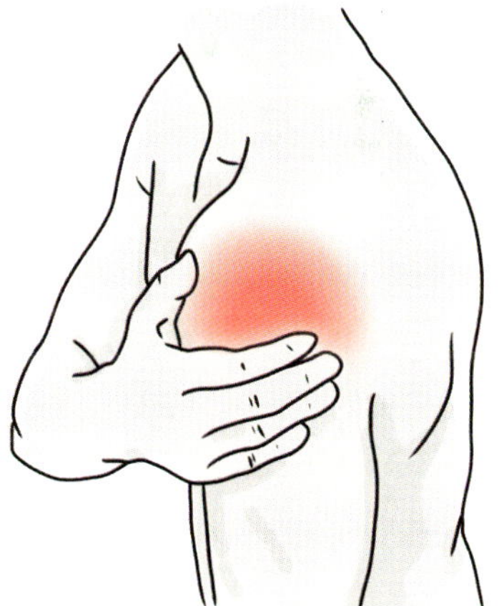

If you don't feel like your pain aligns with either of those causes, there are some other options.

MIDDLE DELTOID PAIN

Most people who come to me thinking that they have an issue with their middle deltoid end up having rotator cuff referral pain. People who truly have an issue with the middle deltoid are usually overdoing dumbbell raises in the gym and not focusing enough on other muscle groups. This places a lot of strain on the deltoids, and it can get to the point where the side of the shoulder becomes tight and painful.

Tree Deltoid Head

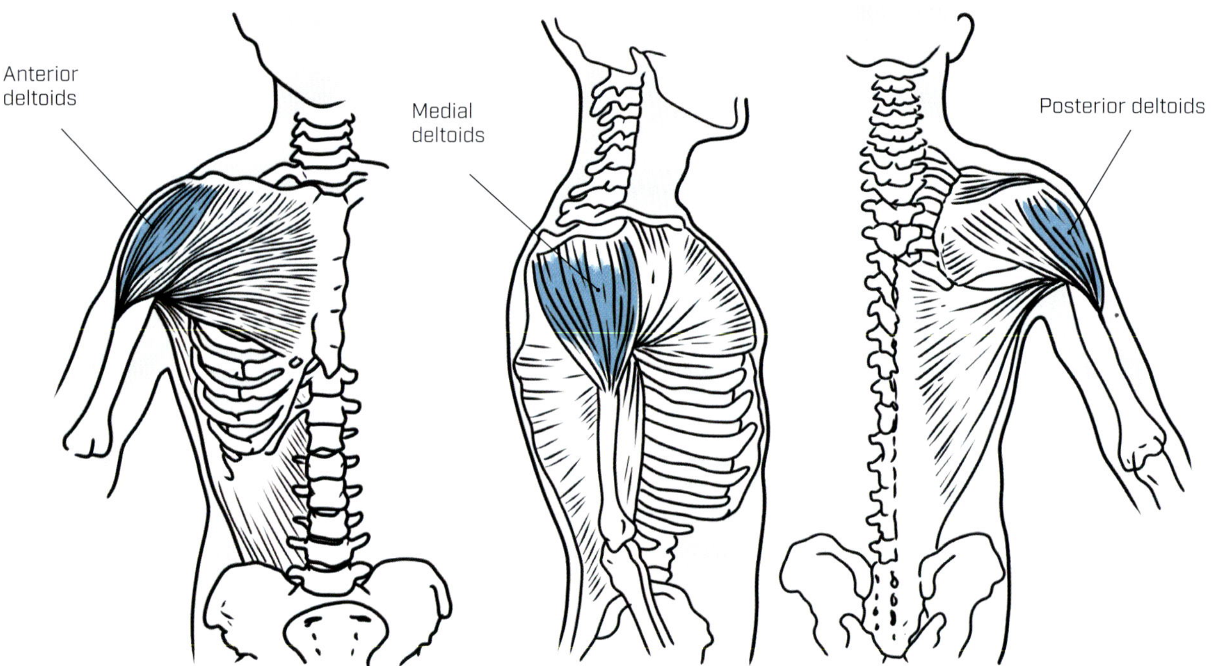

The first step to address deltoid pain is to reduce the weight you are using for dumbbell raises or other weighted overhead movements. Focus on other muscle groups in the back and chest while also making sure you are following all of the advice given in this book for the rotator cuff. Once symptoms reduce, you can slowly start to build back up to the level of exercise you were doing before.

LITTLE LEAGUE SHOULDER

This is a very specific diagnosis seen only in growing kids who play a sport with a lot of overhead movements, like volleyball or softball, but it is most common in young baseball players. This diagnosis refers to a widening in the growth plate in the humerus due to the repeated stress of throwing.

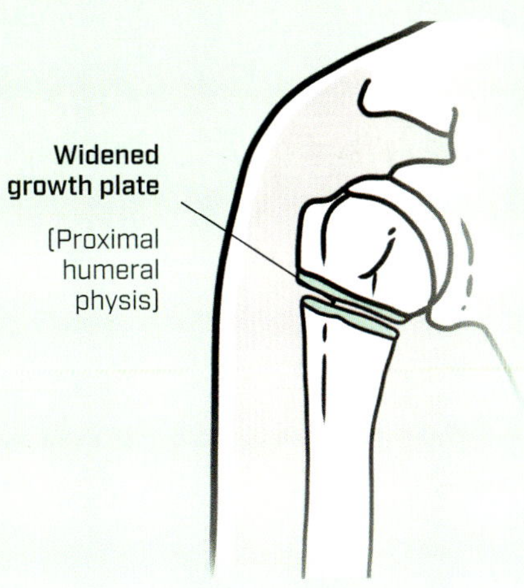

This pain is a deep ache in the middle of the shoulder that worsens when throwing, especially when throwing harder. The only way to properly diagnose it is with an X-ray. If it is confirmed, the athlete will need to take a prolonged break from the sport. The break should include working on the strength of the rotator cuff, which will ultimately make the shoulder significantly stronger for a return to sport. The pain results from the high-velocity movement of throwing or hitting, so exercises will not worsen anything. For a specific timeline for recovery, listen to the individual advice of the overseeing MD and/or PT.

THE BACK OF THE SHOULDER

There are a lot of muscles that lie on the back of the shoulder and can create discomfort but have been covered in other parts of the book:

- Rotator cuff – page 141
- Latissimus dorsi – page 115
- Deltoid – page 152
- Trapezius – page 124
- Triceps – page 162

The muscles that lie between the shoulder blade and the spine are covered in the "Mid Back" section on page 111.

SELF-MASSAGE TECHNIQUE & MOBILITY, FLEXIBILITY, AND STRENGTHENING MOVEMENTS FOR THE SHOULDER

SELF-MASSAGE

The only two things you need to self-massage the important parts of the shoulder are a lacrosse ball and a sturdy wall. (A lacrosse ball truly is the best ball for this—the size and rigidity are perfect.) The most important area to roll out is the "magic triangle" in the back of the shoulder blade where the three rotator cuff muscles lie, specifically the bottom two, the infraspinatus and the teres minor.

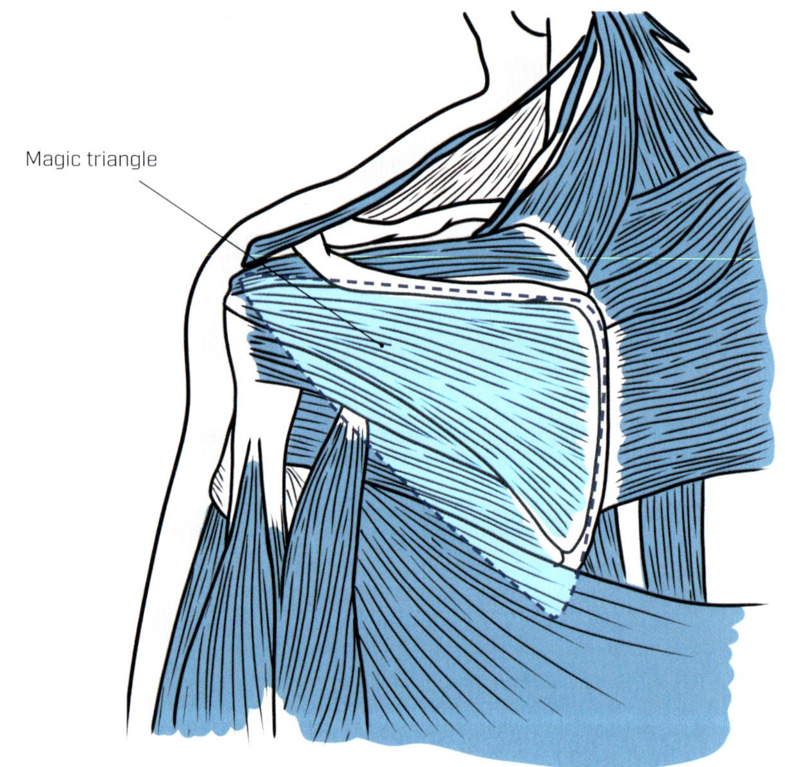

To roll out this area, place a lacrosse ball between your shoulder and the wall and lean your body weight into the ball. Keep the shoulder you are working on as relaxed as possible as you gently shift your weight from side to side looking for tight or tender spots in the musculature. Once you find a tight spot, roll gently for a minute or so before finding other tight spots. Continue for three to five minutes, making sure that when you're done, you feel better than when you started. If you feel sore or bruised afterward, you were probably pressing too hard. Do this before doing the rotator cuff exercises or any upper body exercises.

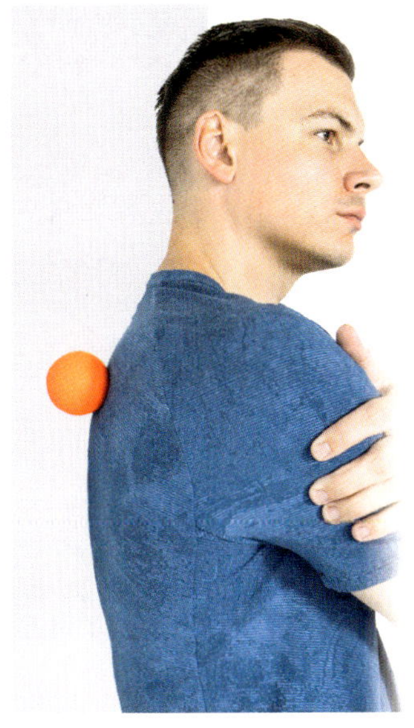

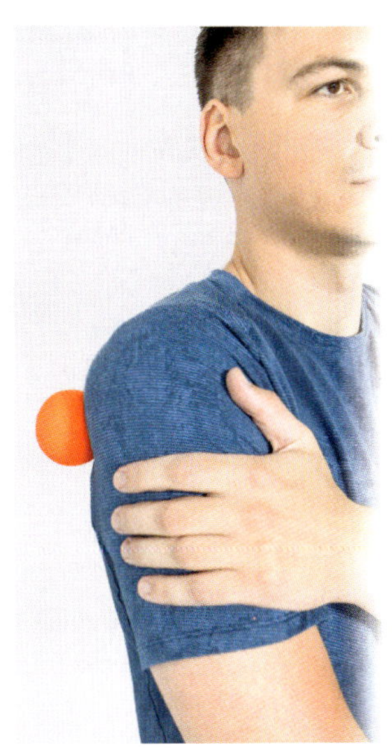

MOBILITY

If you feel pain or tightness when you try to lift your arm above shoulder height, wall slides are the perfect way to address it. Stand facing a wall and place your hand on a towel (to help you slide easily), putting slight pressure on the wall and sliding your hand up the wall while focusing on keeping your shoulder in a down-and-back position. The slight pressure and focus on keeping the shoulder down and back will ensure that you engage the proper muscles. Raise your hand up to the point of comfort and then bring it back down to where you started. When you feel like you can't raise your hand any higher, lean in toward the wall slightly to achieve a slight stretch in the armpit area. Repeat for two sets of ten repetitions, and then stand with your torso turned to a 45-degree angle away from the wall and repeat the same process. As all of the slides become easier, you should notice that it becomes easier to raise your arm overhead without support.

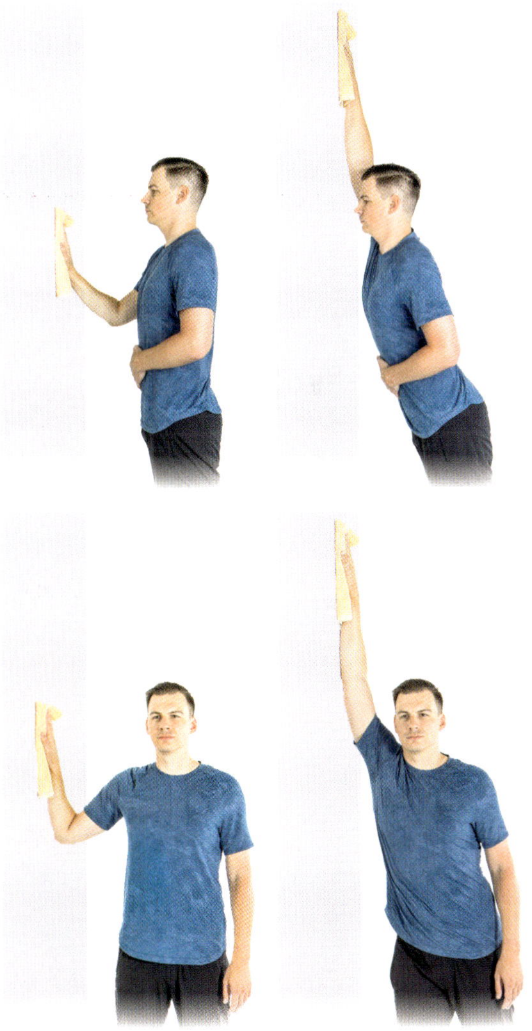

FLEXIBILITY

If you're looking to reduce tightness in the back of your shoulder, stick with the rolling technique described in the "Self-Massage" section. For the front of the shoulder, try these two stretches.

BICEPS STRETCH

Stand in a doorway with your hand and wrist against doorjamb and a slight bend in your elbow. Keep your chest tall as you slowly twist away from the hand. The goal to feel a gentle stretch your biceps and to hold stretch for twenty seconds, three times. Feel free repeat this stretch as needed.

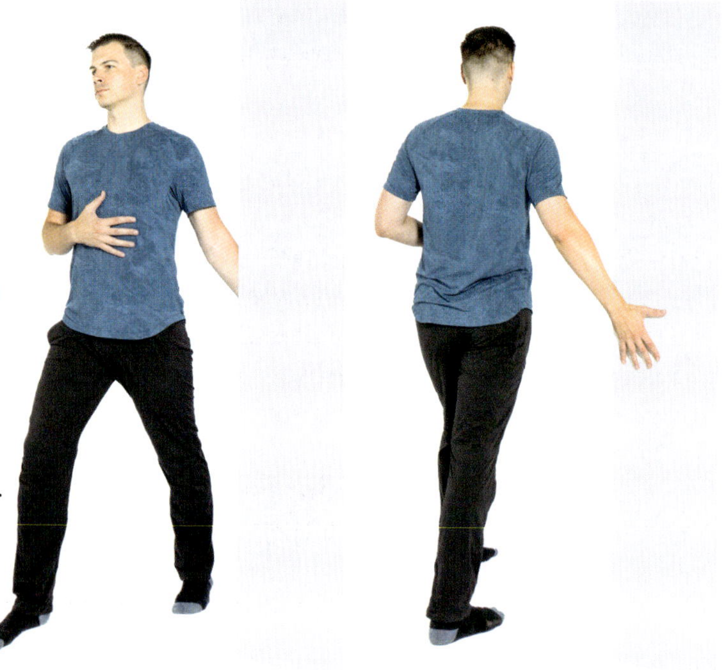

PECTORALIS STRETCH

Stand in a doorway with your arm at shoulder height, your elbow bent at a 90-degree angle, and your forearm pressed against the doorjamb. Keep your chest tall as you slowly twist away from the arm until you feel a gentle stretch in the chest. This stretch should feel gentle and should not aggravate any pain or numbness. Hold the stretch for about twenty seconds and repeat three times.

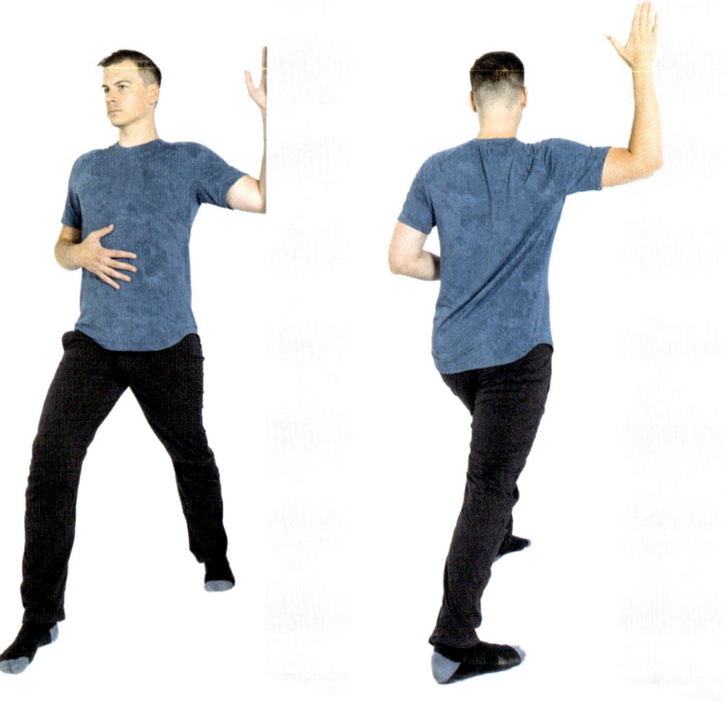

STRENGTHENING

These exercises are the staples that I use to reduce pain and discomfort, including my favorite exercises for the rotator cuff and mid back. If you follow the advice in this book, your discomfort should lessen, and you can begin to do a multitude of other exercises for the upper body. I recommend seeing a physical therapist in person to make sure that you are safely and efficiently expanding the exercises that you do for the upper body.

RESISTED INTERNAL ROTATION

Secure a resistance band to something stable at your elbow height, and bend your elbow to 90 degrees. Start with your hand stretching the band away from your body, keeping your elbow pressed into your torso as you pull the band across your body until your forearm meets your abdomen. Slowly bring your hand back to where it started and repeat for three sets of ten repetitions.

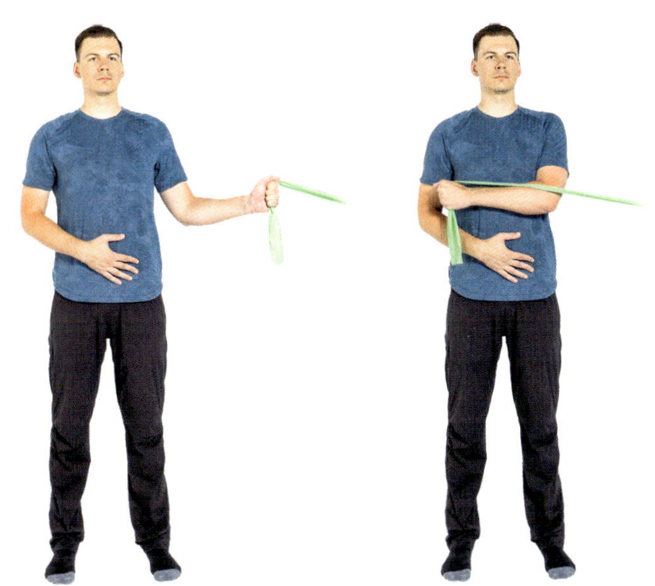

RESISTED EXTERNAL ROTATION

Hold a resistance band with both hands (one end in each hand) while keeping your elbows at a 90-degree angle and pressed into your torso. Keeping your palms facing each other and your elbows pressed into the sides of your torso, slowly bring your hands away from each other against the resistance of the band, then slowly return to the point where you started. Repeat for three sets of ten repetitions.

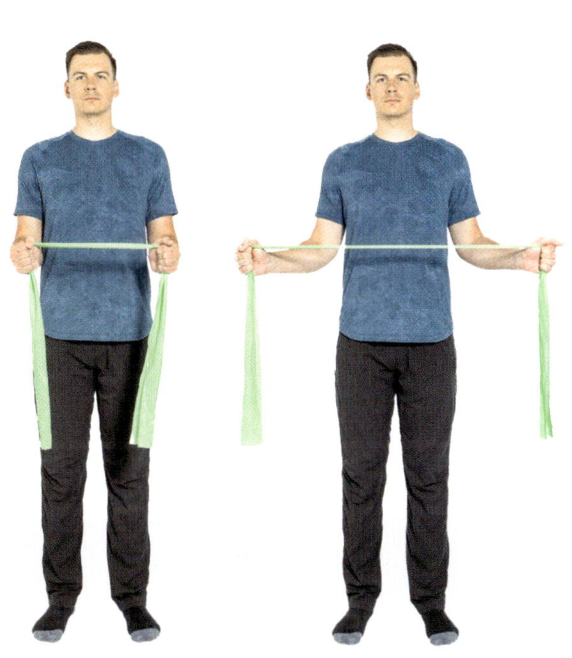

RESISTED EXTERNAL ROTATION ISOMETRIC RAISES

Starting in the same position as the resisted external rotations, pull the resistance band until your hands are just slightly wider than your elbows. Keep your elbows bent at 90 degrees and raise the band to about the level of your forehead without allowing your shoulders to rise. From there, lower your hands back to where they started, then repeat the movement without taking tension away from the band. Keep your hands wider than your elbows throughout the entire movement. Repeat for three sets of six repetitions.

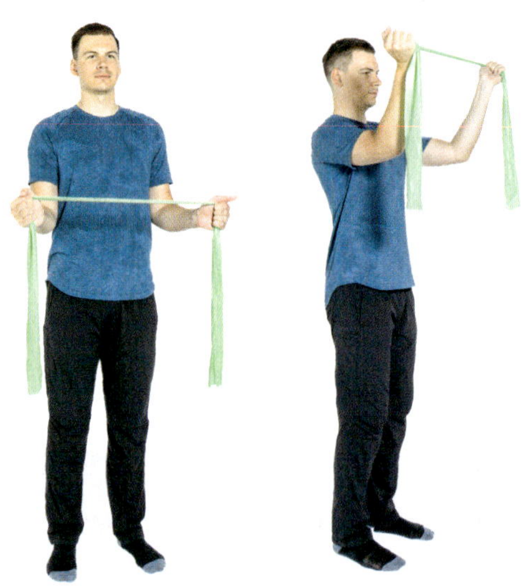

RESISTED PNF D2 FLEXION

Secure one end of the resistance band at your hip. Hold the other end with your opposite hand and imagine you are a pirate about to pull your sword out of its sheath. Keeping your pulling elbow slightly bent, raise that arm at an angle, pulling across your body and against the resistance of the band. At the top of the movement, you should be able to keep your shoulder low despite the fact that your hand is above your head. This movement should feel like your hand and shoulder are being pulled in opposite directions. In the top position, you also want to have that "sword" pointed straight behind you. Slowly return to the starting position by imagining that you are placing the sword back in its sheath. Repeat for three sets of six repetitions.

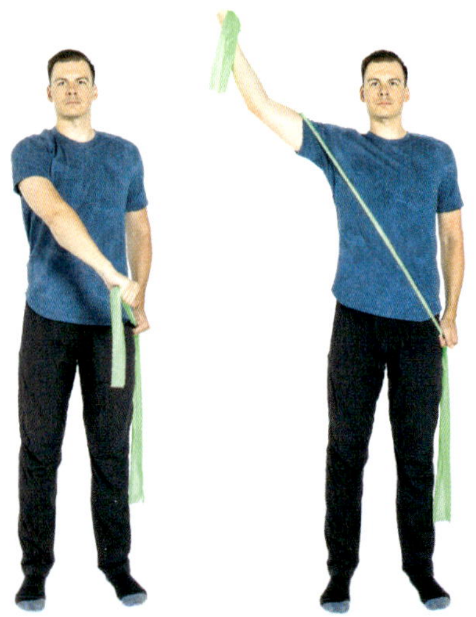

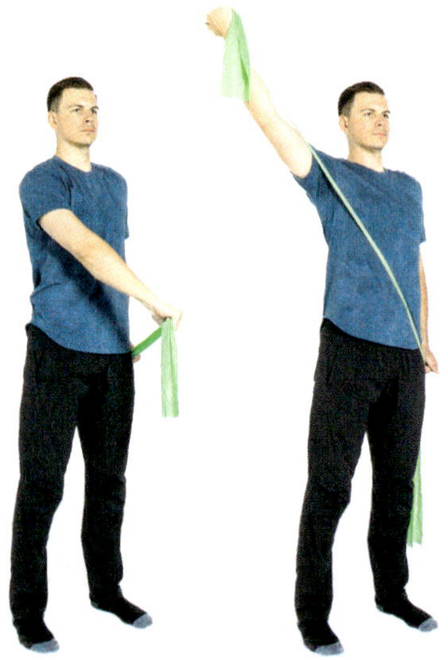

SECTION 7

THE ELBOW AND THE FOREARM

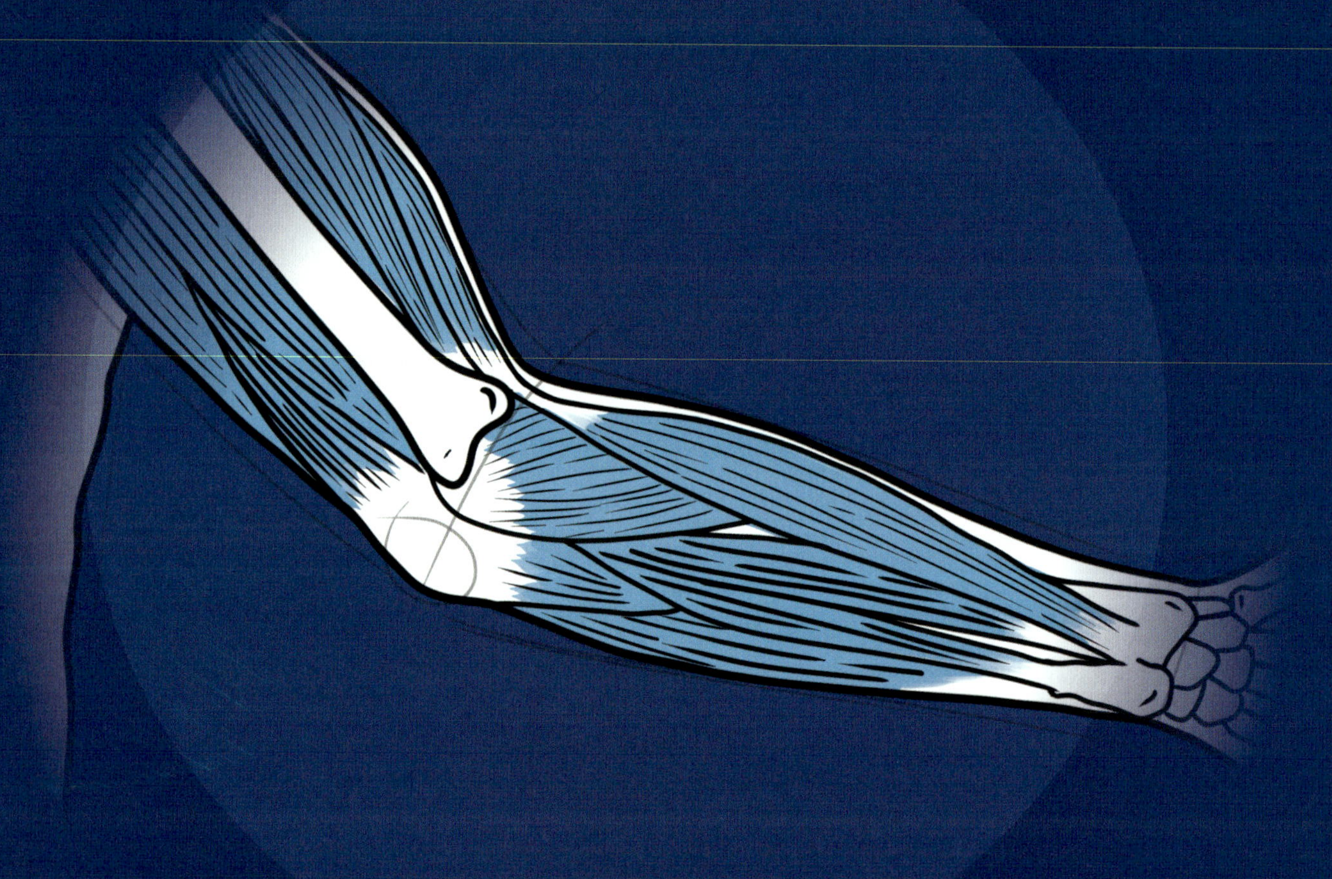

The elbow is one of the simpler joints in the human body, found where the bottom of the humerus meets the tops of the radius and ulna in the lower arm. All of the muscles that end around the elbow start near the shoulder, and most of the muscles that start in the elbow run all the way down the forearm and into the wrist. Because of this anatomical layout, the elbow is somewhat of a passive participant in whatever is happening in the shoulder and the wrist. So, if you're not having success in reducing your elbow pain by following the advice in this chapter, make sure you also dive into the shoulder and wrist sections of this book.

THE FRONT OF THE ELBOW (ELBOW PIT)

BICEPS AND BRACHIALIS PAIN

When you experience pain in the front of the elbow, the two main culprits are the biceps and the brachialis muscles in the upper arm. The biceps originates in the shoulder, and if the irritation is focused in the shoulder joint rather than in the muscle, check "The Shoulder" section of this book (starting on page 141) for advice. But when the biceps muscle is irritated near the elbow, the issue is usually isolated to the biceps muscle itself. The brachialis, a muscle that runs underneath the biceps from a point about halfway down the humerus and attaches near the biceps, may also be the source of discomfort. Since both of these muscles work to bend the elbow, it's not uncommon for them to become tight and irritated together.

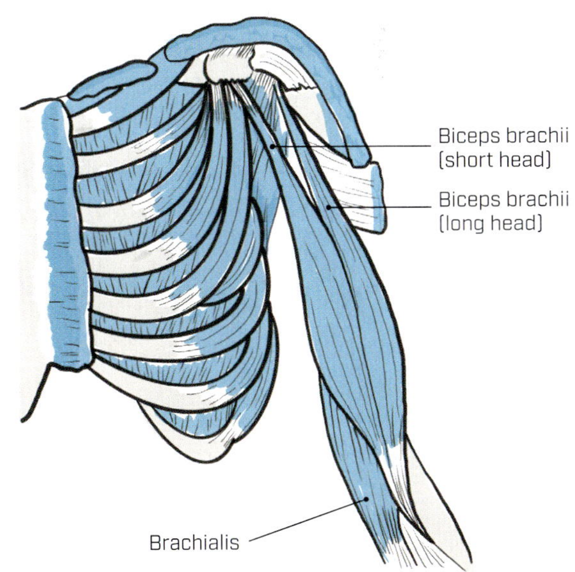

If you overdo biceps curls in the gym or carry and hold heavier objects on a regular basis, you may be familiar with this kind of pain and irritation near the elbow. It may start as a sensation of tightness, but as it progresses, it may become sharper, and you may find the area very tender to the touch. The best first step in resolving the issue is to find and reduce the cause of the symptoms. Then start with the biceps stretch in the shoulder section on page 156, and limit the stress and strain you put on the area. Next, begin to build more strength and control in the muscles by doing light eccentric biceps curls as described on page 171. The lighter weight and the slow and controlled downward motion will help build strength in the muscle and resilience in the tendon, which will ultimately help the pain. This version of a biceps curl is far different from the super heavy and fast-moving biceps curls that are often seen in commercial gyms.

THE BACK OF THE ELBOW (ELBOW BONE)

TRICEPS PAIN

Discomfort on the back of the elbow is caused by tightness or overuse in the triceps muscle, which starts near the shoulder, runs down the back of the arm, and attaches to the bony part of your elbow known as the olecranon process. Pain around this bony attachment can start as tightness but may progress to a sharp pain. You may also find that the area becomes very tender to the touch. This pain can arise if you've been overdoing specific movements such as push-ups but can also occur with the normal activities of daily living.

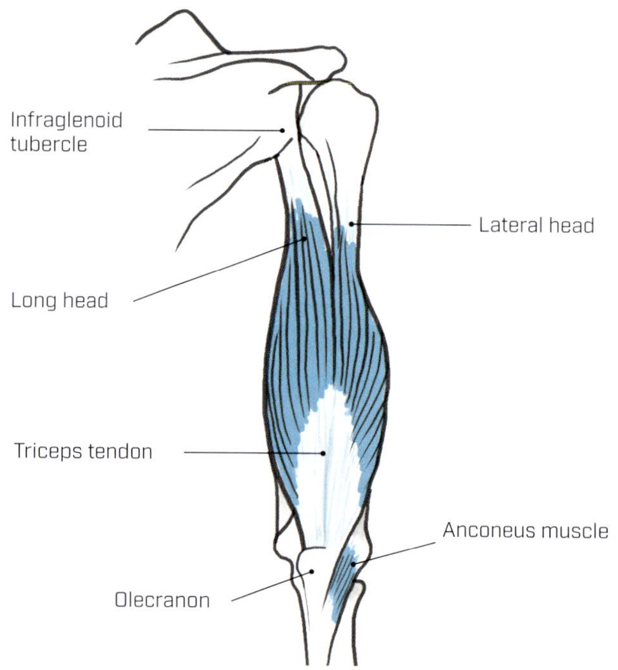

Reducing or eliminating the movement that's causing discomfort while you try to address the tightness in the muscle is the first step to addressing this elbow pain. You can then begin to do the triceps stretch on page 169 and the slow and controlled eccentric triceps pull-downs on page 171. The stretch will improve the flexibility of the muscle, while the exercise will build control of the muscle and resilience in the tendon. Once symptoms reduce, you can then start to build back to all of the normal activities you were doing before.

OLECRANON BURSITIS

Right where the triceps attaches at the olecranon process, you also have a bursa sac that can become inflamed and swollen. As mentioned earlier in the book, a bursa sac is a fluid-filled pouch designed to reduce friction from the tendons. The area may even become slightly warm, red, and painful to the touch. A common cause of pain at the bursa site is direct trauma to the area due to a fall or sustaining a blow on the bony part of the elbow. The best thing to do when this happens is to rest and avoid pressure on the olecranon process. As the symptoms start to reduce, you can begin to do the triceps activities (starting on page 169) to ensure a full recovery.

If swelling and irritation persists despite resting and avoiding pressure to the area, seek out professional guidance.

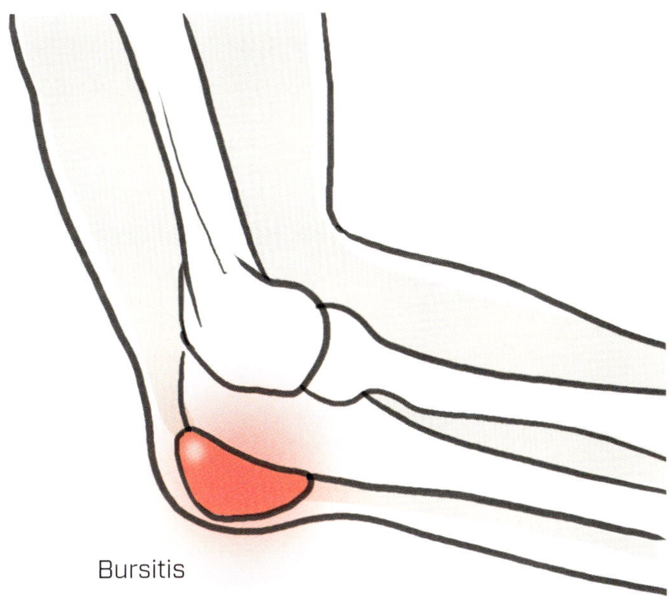

THE TOP OF THE FOREARM AT THE ELBOW

LATERAL EPICONDYLITIS (TENNIS ELBOW)

Tennis elbow gets its name from its prevalence among tennis players who are really focusing on their backhand and overusing the muscle group that extends the wrist. In my practice, I have treated hundreds of cases of "tennis elbow," and not one of the patients has been a tennis player. I see this diagnosis in manual laborers or people who do a lot of work with their hands and in desk workers who type and use a mouse all day. The early symptom of tennis elbow is tightness in the muscles themselves, but it can develop into sharp pain at the lateral epicondyle (the bony protuberance at the elbow end of the humerus), or you may experience pain where the muscles cross the wrist. If you feel a pain in the top of the forearm when using the hand or wrist or when gripping and holding something heavy, you have a textbook case of tennis elbow.

Anytime there are multiple muscles attaching at the same point, there is the possibility for pain and discomfort at that point. The muscles that extend the wrist all attach at the same spot on the top area of the elbow on the lateral epicondyle of the humerus. These muscles extend the wrist and also provide wrist stability.

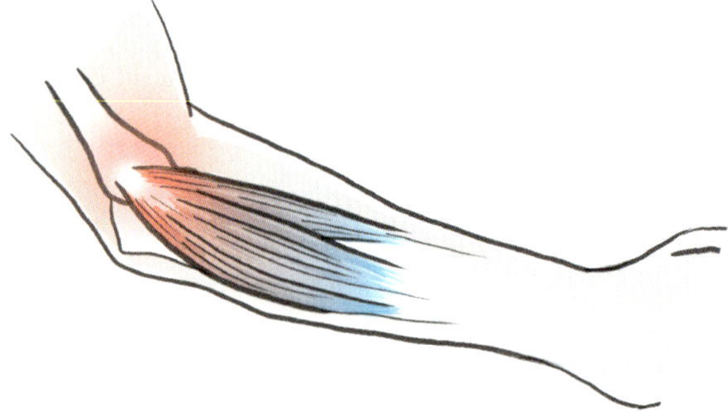

To relieve the symptoms, start by limiting gripping, holding, or anything that provokes your symptoms. You can also administer self-massage to the muscles by following the directions on page 167. Additionally, it is important to do the forearm extensor stretch and the resisted forearm extension exercise on page 170. Applying a mixture of self-massage, stretching, and strengthening techniques to this muscle group on a consistent basis should greatly reduce symptoms.

If you address tennis elbow early, it often begins to clear up quickly. But if you notice that the symptoms are stubborn, it is a good idea to see your friendly neighborhood PT for more advanced manual therapy techniques.

THE BOTTOM OF THE FOREARM AT THE ELBOW

MEDIAL EPICONDYLITIS (GOLFER'S ELBOW)

Golfer's elbow is far less common than its counterpart on the top of the forearm, tennis elbow, but it has a very similar presentation. Tightness and irritation develop in the wrist flexor muscles on the bottom side of the forearm that originate at the medial epicondyle of the humerus and run down and cross the wrist. Heavy lifting, gripping, carrying, or gripping and swinging something like a golf club can cause symptoms.

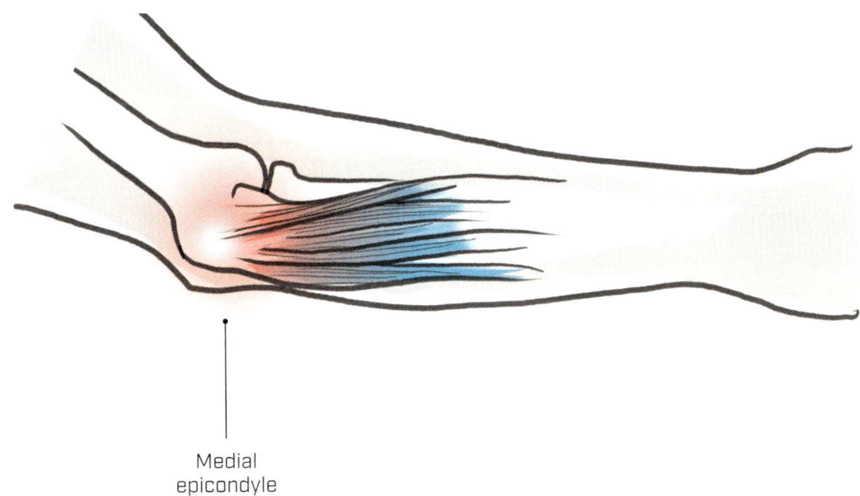

Tightness in this muscle group can develop into sharp pain right over the medial epicondyle, at the elbow, or it might extend to the wrist. Reducing the workload on the muscles for a couple of weeks will help with the symptoms. You can also do the wrist flexor stretch a few times a day and the wrist flexion exercise once a day (see pages 168 and 169). Applying the self-massage techniques for the wrist flexors (see page 167) in addition to the exercises should hopefully be all you need to reduce symptoms in this area.

CUBITAL TUNNEL SYNDROME

If what you're feeling in this area of the elbow is less of a tightness or pain and more of a numbness or tingling, then you may be experiencing cubital tunnel syndrome. The cubital tunnel is also known as the "funny bone." If you've ever hit this spot on your elbow just right, you know how painful it can be with just an edge of ticklishness. Cubital tunnel syndrome presents with similar symptoms, but it lingers. It is essentially an impingement of the ulnar nerve where it passes through the forearm. The cubital tunnel, where the ulnar nerve is located, is vulnerable because it basically allows direct access to the nerve. It doesn't take much of a bump or a lot of compression to create symptoms.

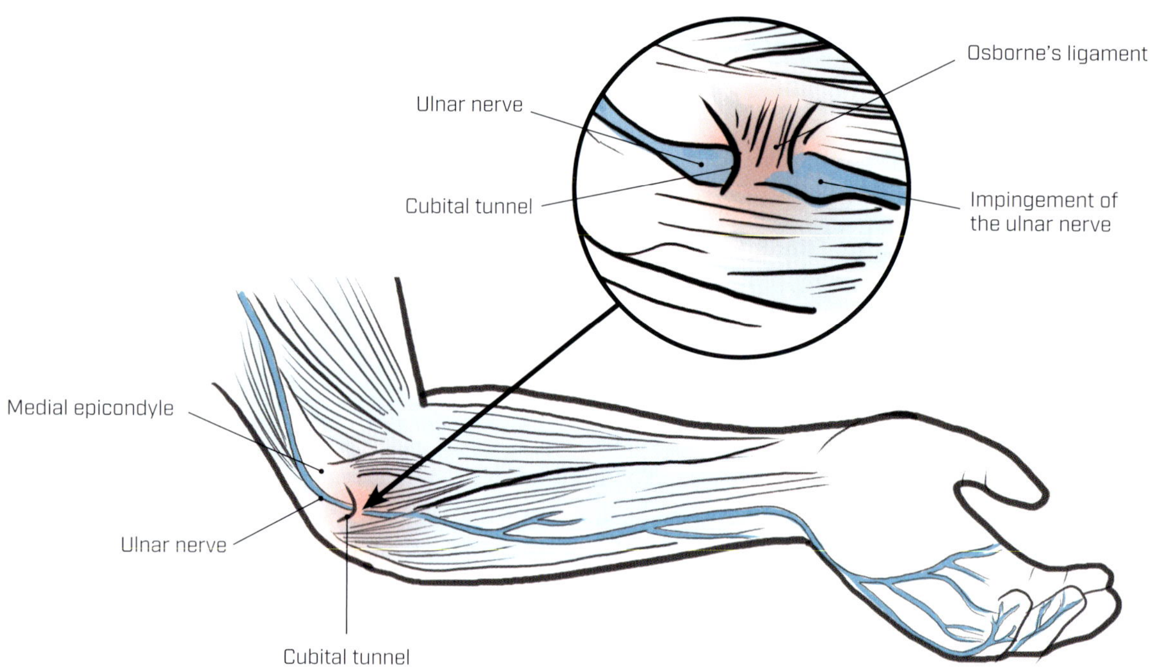

While it is helpful to follow the advice for golfer's elbow on page 165 to ensure the muscles in the area are as flexible and strong as possible, you will receive the most relief from the ulnar nerve glides found on page 168. Doing these gently throughout the day will help to desensitize the nerve and allow for more pain-free movement in the elbow. Limit pressure or compression at the elbow as much as you can while you heal.

SELF-MASSAGE TECHNIQUES & MOBILITY, FLEXIBILITY, AND STRENGTHENING MOVEMENTS FOR THE ELBOW AND FOREARM

SELF-MASSAGE

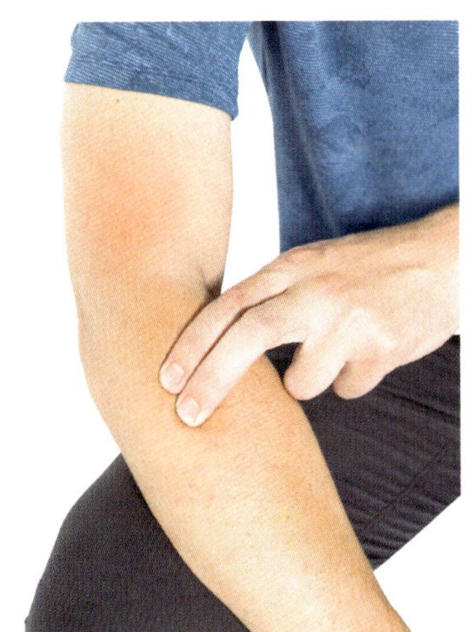

WRIST EXTENSORS

Seated with the forearm you would like to massage resting on a sturdy surface in front of you, take your first two fingers of the other hand and locate the forearm extensor muscle group. You can do this by finding the bony prominence of the lateral epicondyle and going down two to three inches until you feel musculature. Use your first two fingers to find tight or tender areas and massage with small circles using a medium pressure. Continue for three to five minutes or until you feel a reduction in tension and symptoms. A gentle setting on a massage gun also works great in this area. Feel free to repeat as necessary.

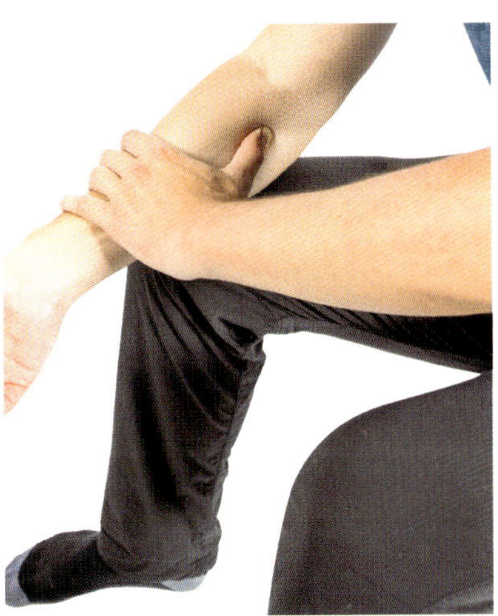

WRIST FLEXORS

Seated with the hand of the forearm you want to massage resting in your lap, take the thumb of your opposite hand and locate the forearm flexor muscle group. You can do this by finding the bony prominence of the medial epicondyle and going down two to three inches. With a firm yet gentle pressure, take your thumb and massage over tight or tender spots you find in the muscle group. Do this for three to five minutes or until you feel a reduction in symptoms. A gentle setting on a massage gun also works well in this area. Repeat as necessary.

MOBILITY

ULNAR NERVE GLIDES

Sitting or standing up straight, take the arm you want to mobilize and hold it out to the side at shoulder height with the elbow bent at ninety degrees. Make the "OK" sign with your thumb and index finger and slowly try to bring your pinky to the outside corner of your eye. Stop when you feel a gentle pull or sensation in the inside of the elbow and return to the starting position. Repeat for two sets of ten multiple times throughout the day, making sure that you are doing them gently enough that you don't increase any symptoms. If you are doing these right, you should notice that they become much easier over time.

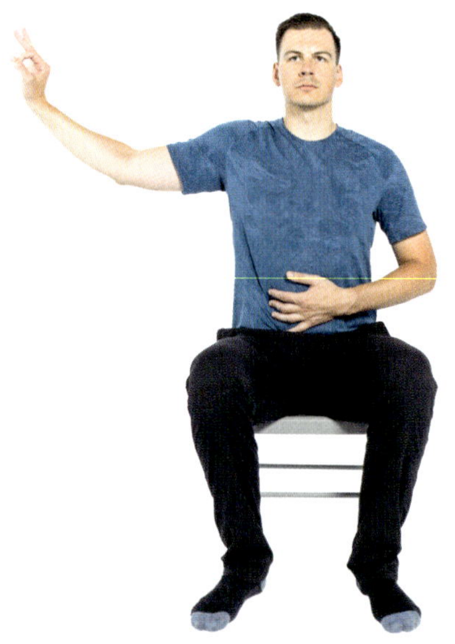

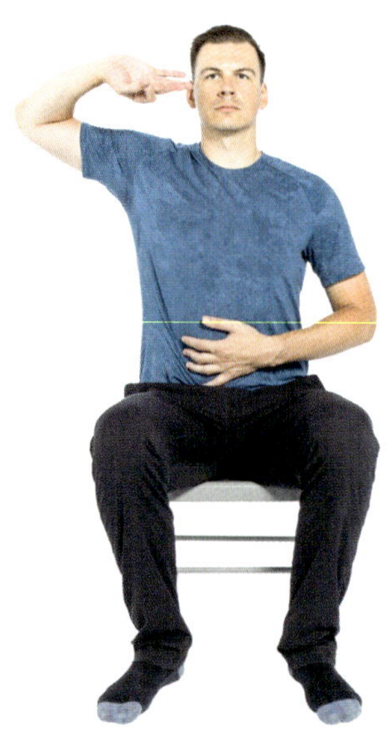

FLEXIBILITY

WRIST EXTENSOR STRETCH

Sit and hold the arm you intend to stretch straight out in front of you with your palm down. Take your opposite hand and pull down on the hand of the arm you are stretching until you feel a slight stretch in the top of your forearm. Once you feel the stretch, hold for twenty seconds and repeat two to three times. You can repeat these steps a few times per day.

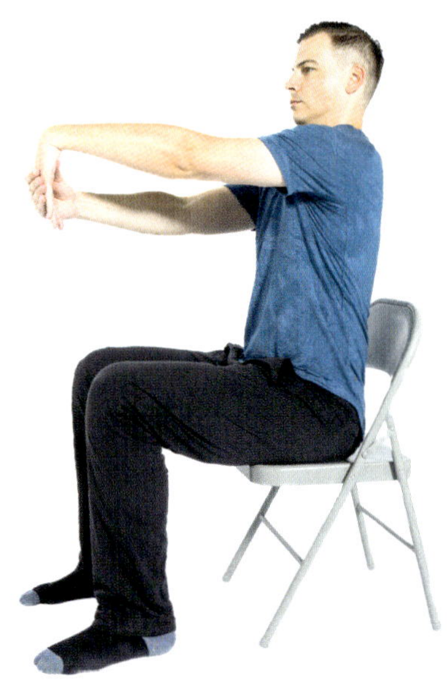

WRIST FLEXOR STRETCH

Sit and hold the arm you intend to stretch straight out in front of you with your palm up. Take your opposite hand and pull down the hand of the arm you are stretching until you feel a stretch on the bottom of the forearm. Once you feel the stretch, hold for twenty seconds and repeat two to three times. Repeat these steps multiple times throughout the day.

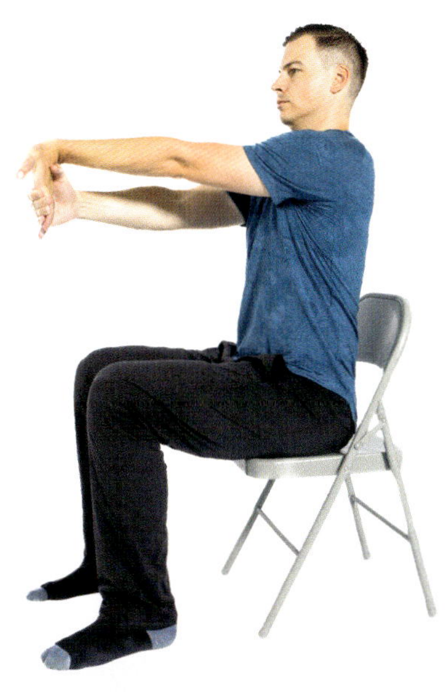

TRICEPS STRETCH

Sitting up straight, take the hand of the arm you intend to stretch and try to place it in between your shoulder blades by reaching over your head. Then take your other hand, grab the elbow of the arm you are stretching, and pull it toward the opposite arm. Stop once you feel a gentle stretch in the back of the arm, then hold for about twenty seconds and repeat two to three times. Repeat this stretch as necessary.

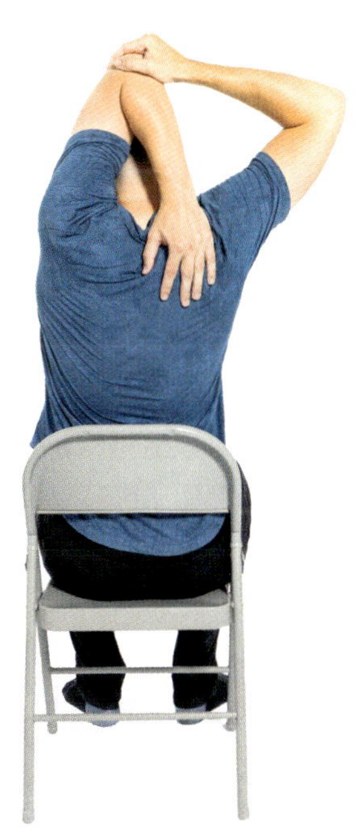

STRENGTHENING

RESISTED WRIST FLEXION

Sit with your forearm resting on your leg and your palm up. Holding onto a resistance band that you secure under your foot, slowly allow your hand to lower as far as it can go before curling it up as far as it can go, then return to the starting position. Repeat for three sets of ten.

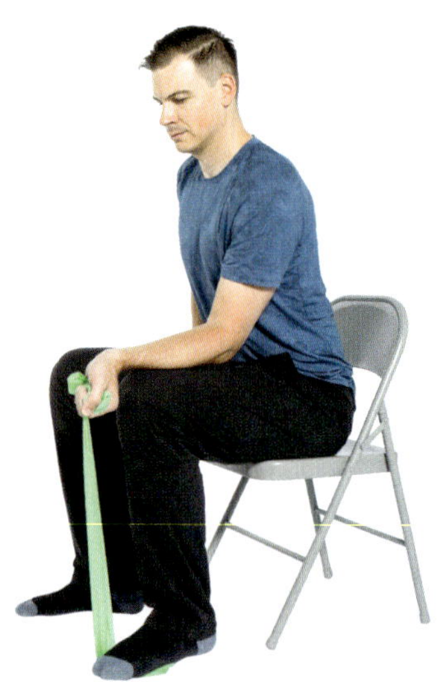

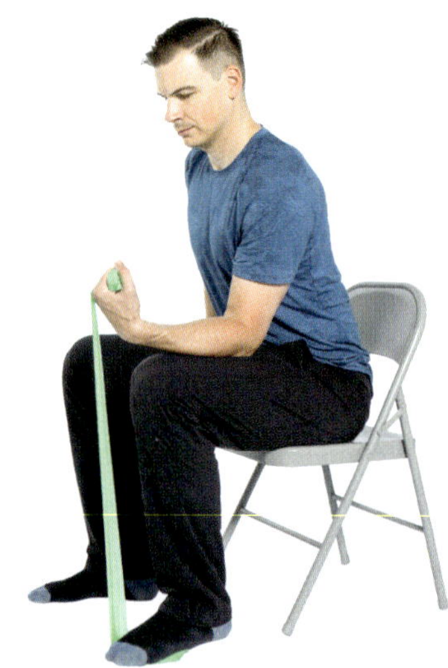

RESISTED WRIST EXTENSION

Sit with your forearm resting on your leg and your palm down. Hold a resistance band in your hand, securing the other end under your foot. Lower your hand as far as it can go, then slowly lift it as far as you can before returning to the starting position. Repeat for three sets of ten.

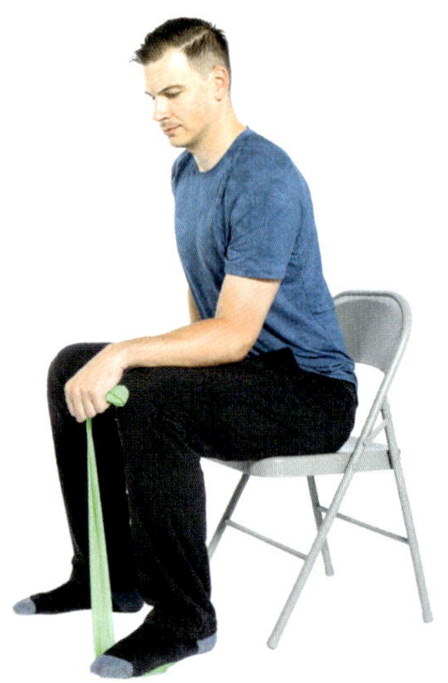

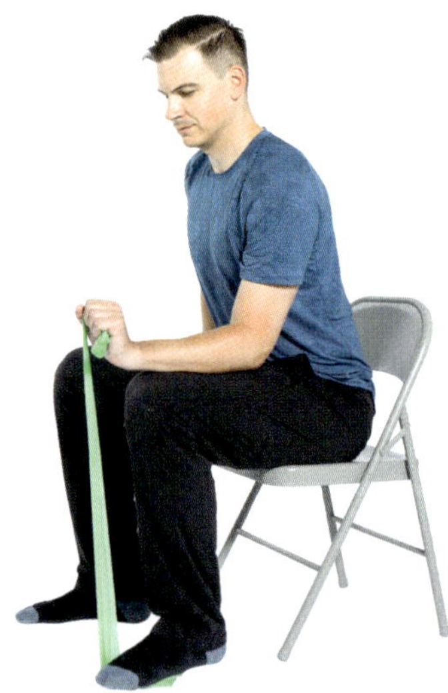

ECCENTRIC BICEPS CURLS

Stand and hold a resistance band in both hands, securing the other end on the floor under your feet. Keeping your arms close to your torso, start from a straight-arm position and then bend your elbows, raising your hands toward your chest against the resistance of the band. Once you can't bring your hands up any further, slowly lower them back to the starting position, taking at least five full seconds to get there. Repeat this for three sets of ten.

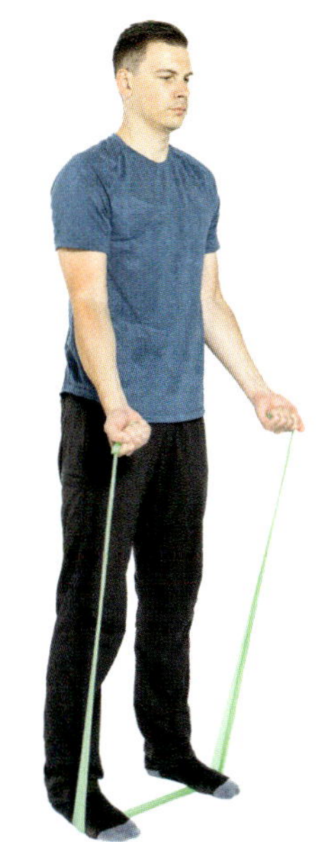

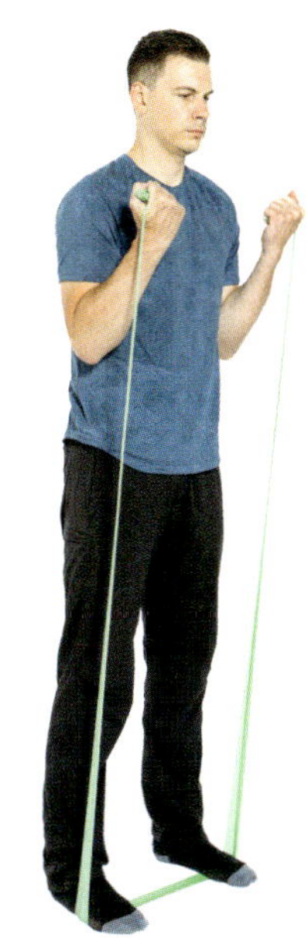

ECCENTRIC TRICEPS PULL-DOWNS

Secure a resistance band above you using a doorway or another sturdy object. Hold onto the band with your palms facing down. Keeping your arms against your torso, push your hands toward the floor against the resistance of the band. Once your arms are as straight as you can make them, slowly raise your hands back to the starting position, taking at least five full seconds to get there. Repeat this for three sets of ten.

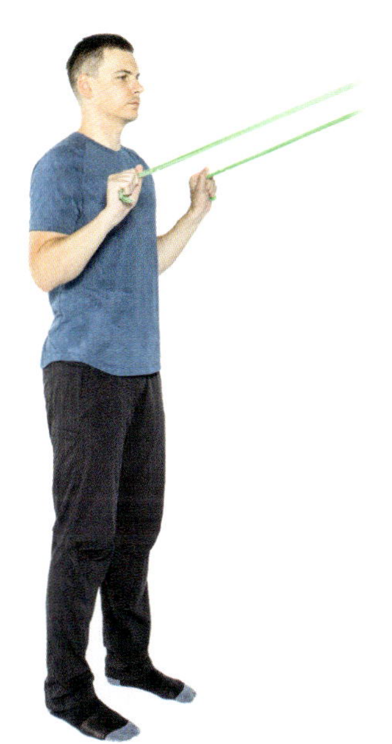

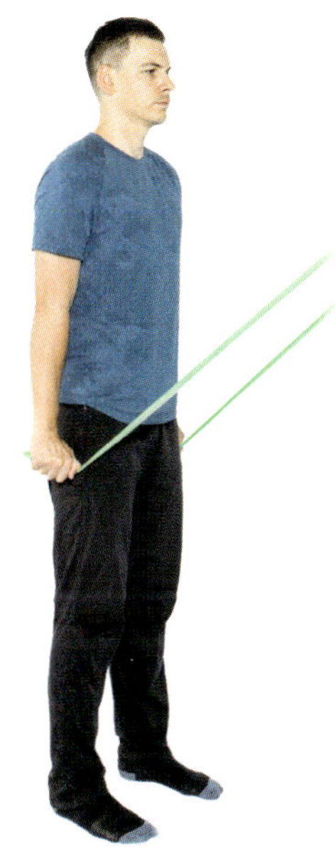

SECTION 8

THE WRIST AND THE HAND

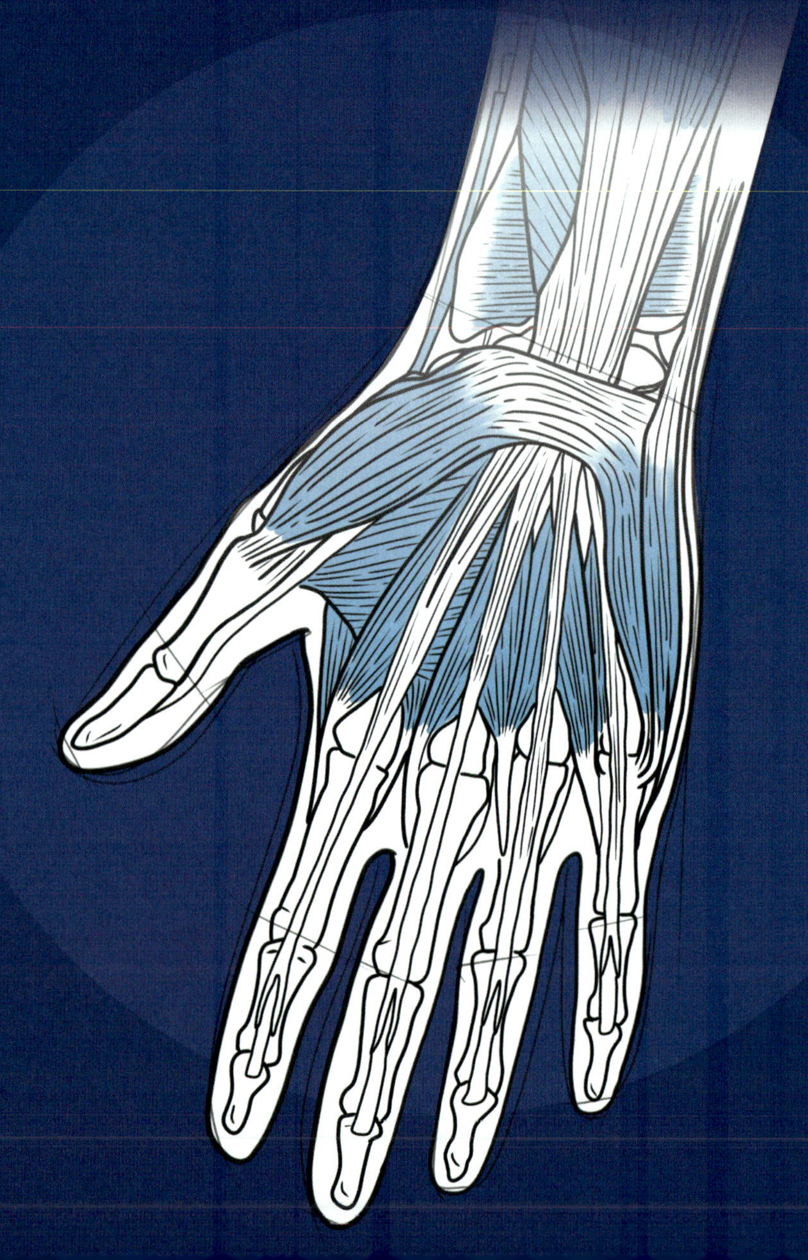

Look at the anatomy of the wrist and hand. All of the tendons that cross the wrist originate in muscles in the forearm and extend into the hand to make it function. When I see a patient with wrist or hand pain, I first look at the forearm and the elbow. In a lot of cases, focusing purely on the muscles of the forearm can fully alleviate pain in the wrist. If the pain is on the top side of the wrist, taking a look at the section on tennis elbow (see page 164) may be the answer. If you're feeling pain on the bottom side of the wrist, make sure to read through the section on golfer's elbow (see page 165) for the same reason.

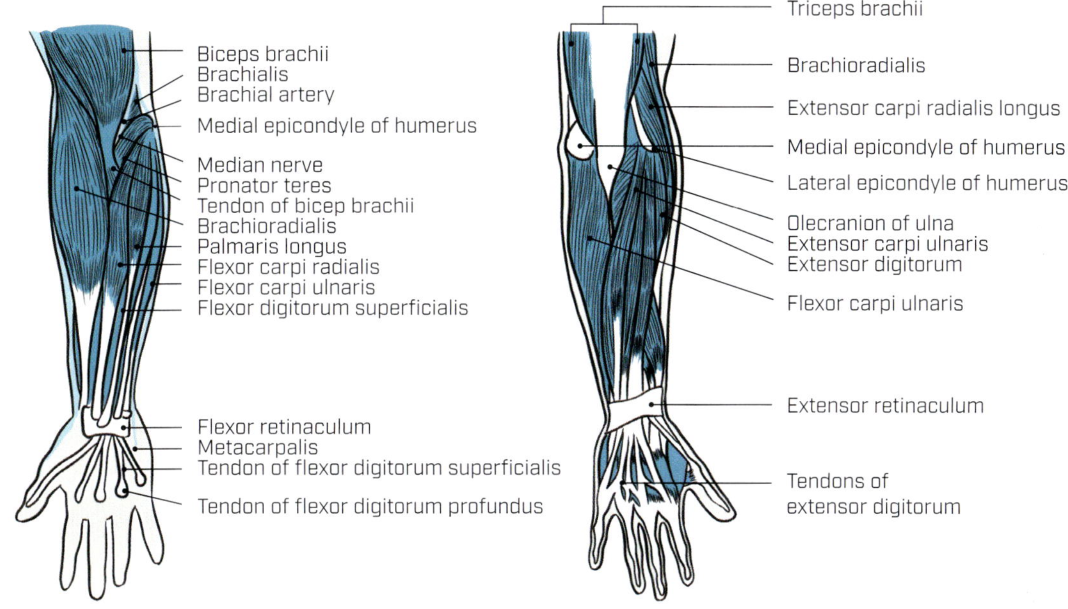

Weakness or tightness on the top or bottom of the wrist may be best addressed through the strengthening and flexibility exercises in *The Forearm and the Elbow* (starting on page 167), and if you're experiencing numbness in the wrist or hand, it's still a good idea to start further up the chain. For the most part, when something is being impinged, it is happening further up the arm or where a structure originates in the neck at the cervical spine or the thoracic outlet (see "The Head, the Neck, and the Jaw, starting on page 123). Especially if your whole hand is going numb or if the numbness extends up the forearm, it is likely coming from one of those areas.

No matter where your numbness comes from, nerve glides can help reduce your symptoms. Numbness mainly in the pinky and outside of the hand is attributed to the ulnar nerve, numbness in the middle and index fingers is likely coming from the median nerve, and numbness mainly in the thumb region is likely the radial nerve. Try the ulnar nerve glides (page 168), median nerve glides (page 180), or radial nerve glides (page 180), depending on your symptoms.

Pain and weakness in the wrist and hand may also have other specific diagnoses, and the following descriptions and exercises may help with your symptoms. As always, if your injury or symptoms persist, seek professional care.

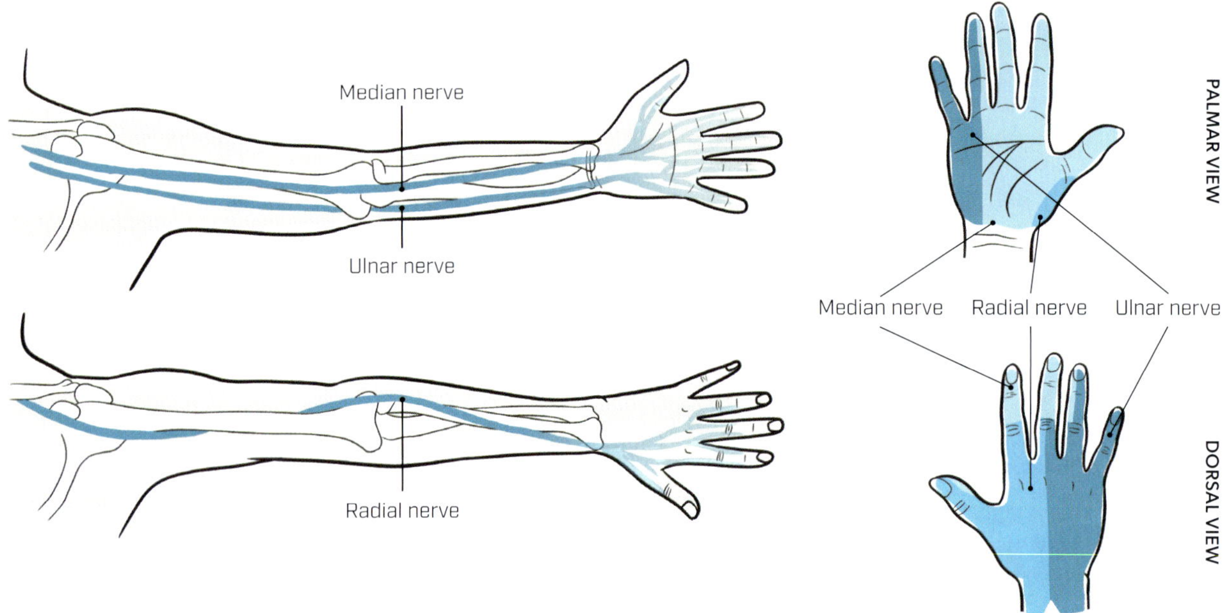

CARPAL TUNNEL SYNDROME

If you still have numbness in the median nerve after trying to address its sources further up the chain, you may have an impingement in the carpal tunnel. The carpal tunnel is a space in the wrist where the median nerve passes into the hand. If there is compression in the area, it can lead to numbness, weakness, and pain in the hand.

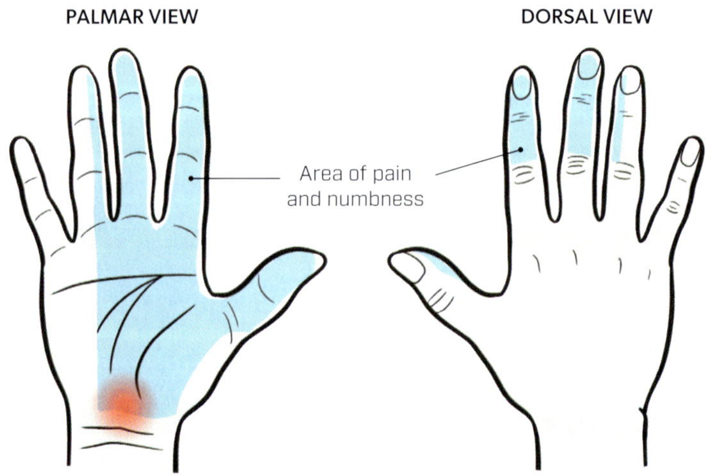

Carpal tunnel syndrome is most commonly an overuse injury. Manual laborers and corporate keyboard warriors alike may find that repetitive use of their hands can create swelling and irritation. Other common causes are previous fractures, other injuries to the wrist, or direct compression over the carpal tunnel itself for prolonged periods of time.

No matter the cause, the forearm stretches on page 169 and the median nerve glides on page 180 may provide some relief. Do these movements frequently throughout the day, along with taking small and frequent breaks from any repetitive tasks.

It is also important to remove anything from your work set-up that might be compressing the area. The wrist cushion for your keyboard might feel nice and supportive at first, but it is actually compressing the carpal tunnel and will lead to symptoms over time. Remove it if you can.

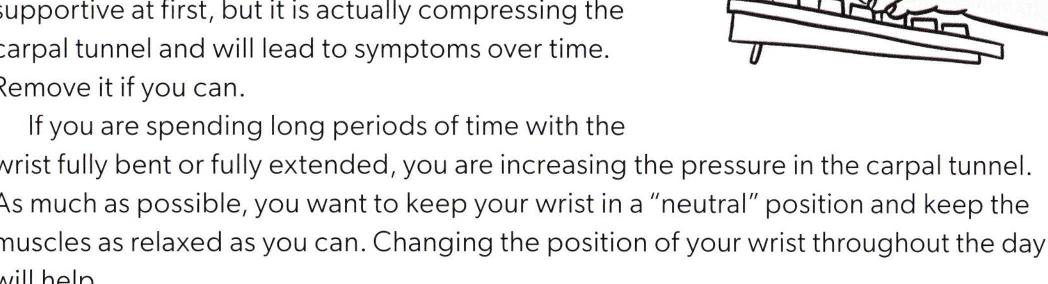

If you are spending long periods of time with the wrist fully bent or fully extended, you are increasing the pressure in the carpal tunnel. As much as possible, you want to keep your wrist in a "neutral" position and keep the muscles as relaxed as you can. Changing the position of your wrist throughout the day will help.

If you're a manual laborer, take more breaks and reduce the tension and pressure you're using when gripping and holding. If you work at a desk all day, try to keep your forearms fully supported and relaxed on the desk in front of you.

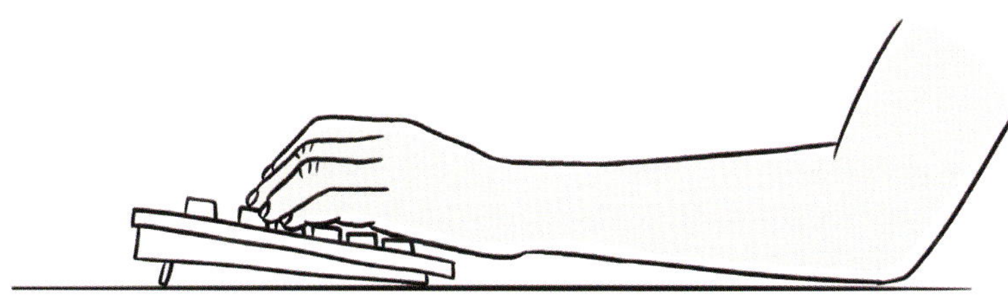

As symptoms reduce, the final step is to build strength in the muscles of the hand and forearm. You can find the forearm exercises on page 170 and the hand exercises on pages 181 and 182. Make sure to start slowly and never irritate your symptoms. The goal is to do the exercises in a way where you feel muscular fatigue but no increased irritation of the numbness or pain.

JOINT PAIN

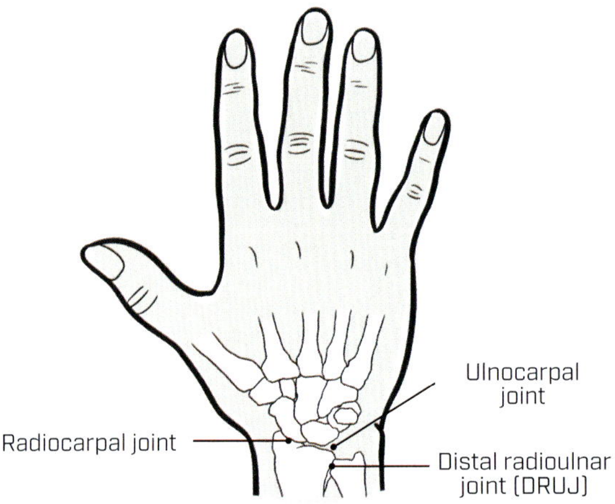

There are three main joints in the wrist: The distal radioulnar joint is where the radius and ulna join together, and the radiocarpal and ulnocarpal joints are where the radius and ulna meet the carpal bones in the hand. Pain in the joint is most common after an injury such as falling forward and landing on an outstretched arm. The joint can also become irritated through overuse or due to arthritis.

If symptoms increase when putting pressure on the wrist through weight-bearing exercises, like a plank position or push-ups, try to keep as much of your weight as possible on the "heel" of your hand to allow your forearm to handle most of the stress. The more weight that shifts toward the fingers, the more stress goes through the joint of the wrist. If shifting weight to the "heel" of the hand isn't enough to reduce symptoms, try taking a break from symptom-provoking movements for one to two weeks.

It's also a good idea to avoid positions where the wrist is fully bent or fully extended. Try to keep the wrist in a neutral position as much as you can to avoid compressing the joint. (See the illustration on page 175.)

As symptoms reduce, you can improve the flexibility of the wrist by following the self-massage and stretching techniques in "The Elbow and the Forearm" starting on page 167. If the stretches irritate your wrist pain, focus on the self-massage techniques until you can do the stretches pain free. You can also focus on the wrist mobilization found on page 168 to directly increase the mobility of the wrist and improve its ability to bear weight.

Finally, the stronger the muscles of the forearm and hand are, the more stress you will take off the wrist joint itself. Focusing on the forearm and hand exercises found on pages 179 to 182 will help the wrist in the long term.

TRIANGULAR FIBROCARTILAGE COMPLEX [TFCC] SPRAIN

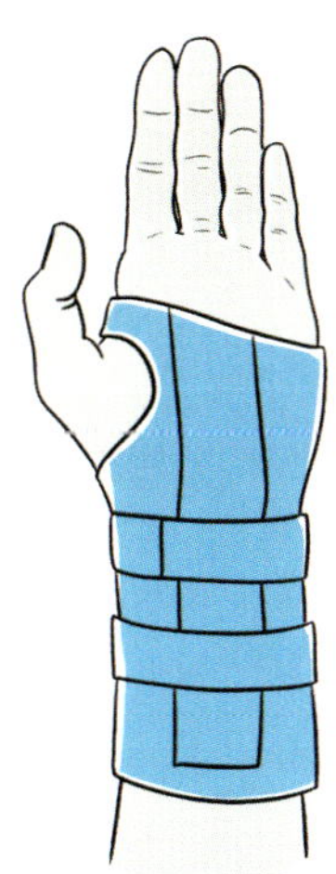

If you have pain on the pinky side of your wrist when doing movements like a push-up or bench press, you may have a TFCC sprain or small tear. The most common cause of this injury is a traumatic event like falling on an outstretched hand, but it may be caused by repetitive overuse. Your wrist will generally feel okay until you try to put weight on it.

If your symptoms are minimal, wearing a specific TFCC brace can reduce the pain while allowing you to continue normal wrist and hand movements. If the brace isn't enough, then it is a good idea to seek medical help. You may need an X-ray or MRI to assess the level of damage to the area and determine if long-term immobilization or surgery is needed.

Once the injury has had a chance to heal, you can start to follow the advice for joint pain on the previous page (176).

DE QUERVAIN'S TENOSYNOVITIS

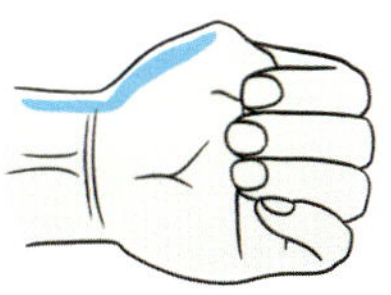

If you're feeling pain in the area where the thumb meets the wrist, then you might be dealing with De Quervain's Tenosynovitis. If you make a fist with your thumb tucked under your other fingers and feel a significant increase in pain as you tilt your wrist toward the pinky, you likely have inflammation in that area caused by a recent and significant increase in how often you are using your hands.

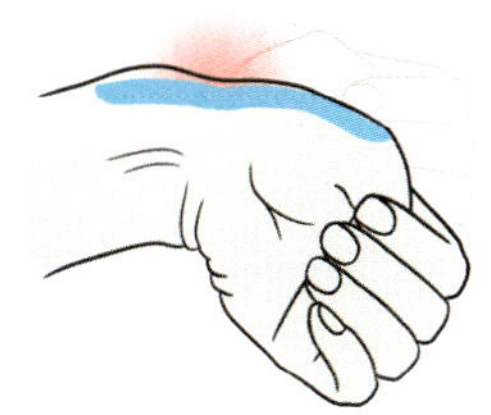

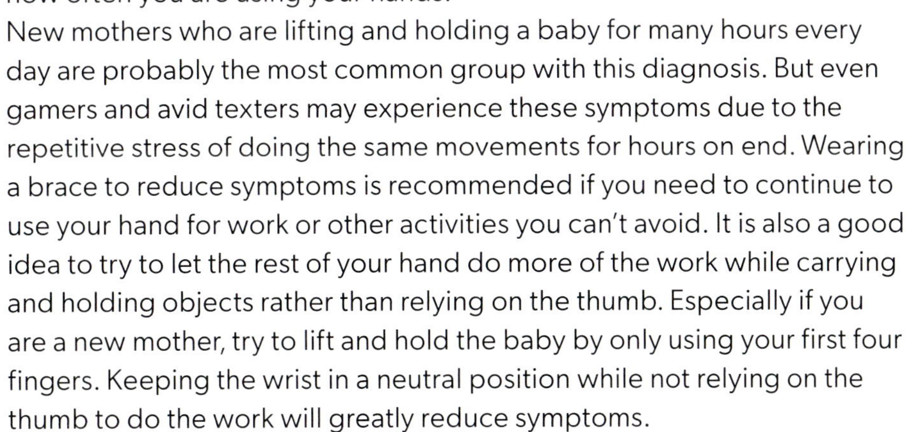

New mothers who are lifting and holding a baby for many hours every day are probably the most common group with this diagnosis. But even gamers and avid texters may experience these symptoms due to the repetitive stress of doing the same movements for hours on end. Wearing a brace to reduce symptoms is recommended if you need to continue to use your hand for work or other activities you can't avoid. It is also a good idea to try to let the rest of your hand do more of the work while carrying and holding objects rather than relying on the thumb. Especially if you are a new mother, try to lift and hold the baby by only using your first four fingers. Keeping the wrist in a neutral position while not relying on the thumb to do the work will greatly reduce symptoms.

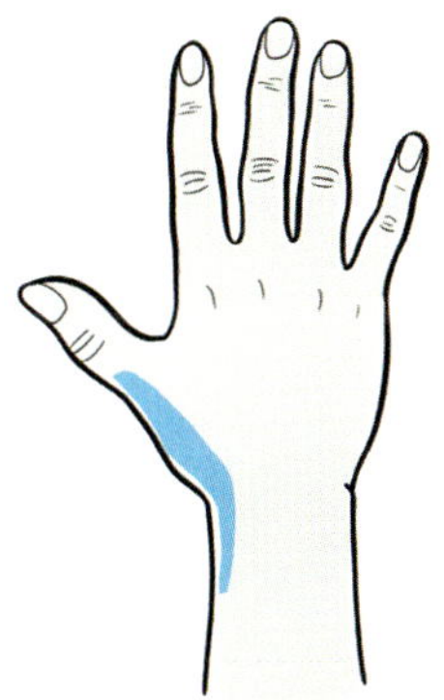

As the symptoms decrease, you can start to do the wrist and hand exercises found at the end of this section. Building strength and flexibility throughout the entire wrist and hand will help to take away further stress from this area.

POLLICIS TENDON/MUSCLE PAIN

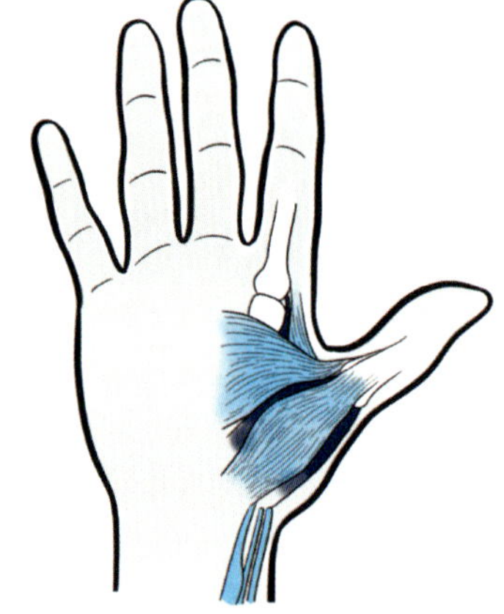

If your pain is more significant on the palm side of the thumb, you may be suffering from overuse in the pollicis muscles themselves. Found in the "thumb pad," the pollicis muscles control the thumb. Massaging that area directly can reduce symptoms (see page 179).

The thumb exercise on page 182 can also help. It is a good idea to reduce strain in the thumb by reducing the movements you are doing with your thumbs. Taking frequent breaks to do the self-massage and exercise while also trying to use your hand and forearm to do more of the work of gripping and holding is advised.

Over time, this muscle group should become stronger and more flexible through exercise, resulting in a decrease in symptoms.

THE DIGITS

If you are having pain in the other four fingers that doesn't align with carpal tunnel or the other nerve-related diagnoses listed in this section, focus on the flexibility and strength of the muscles in the forearm, which is where most of the muscles that control the fingers are located.

If you are having longstanding finger pain that isn't responding to the techniques in this book, find an occupational therapist (OT) who is a certified hand specialist (CHT) to help you. OTs, not PTs, are the specialists when it comes to treating the hands and fingers.

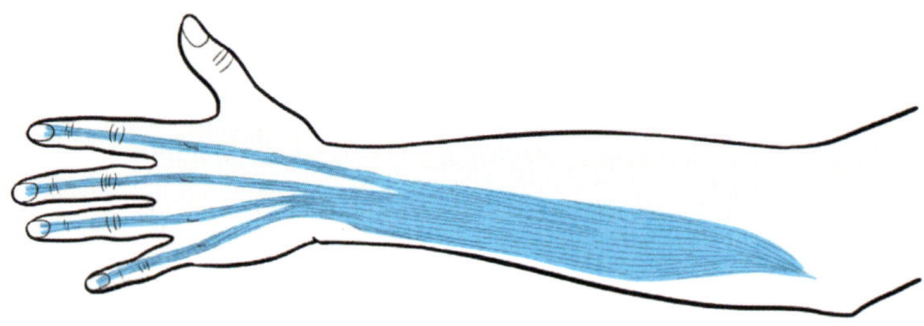

SELF-MASSAGE TECHNIQUES & MOBILITY AND STRENGTHENING MOVEMENTS FOR THE WRIST AND HAND

SELF-MASSAGE

POLLICIS MUSCLES (THE THUMB PAD)

Make a fist with your opposite hand and press the knuckles of your first two fingers and into the thumb pad of the hand you want to work on. Keep the hand completely relaxed while you find the tight and tender areas of the muscle with your other knuckles. Use a medium pressure and focus on areas of the thumb where you feel especially tight. Massage those areas for three to five minutes and repeat as necessary. You should feel some relief immediately, but if you feel more soreness after the massage, then you used pressure that was too deep, or you went for too long.

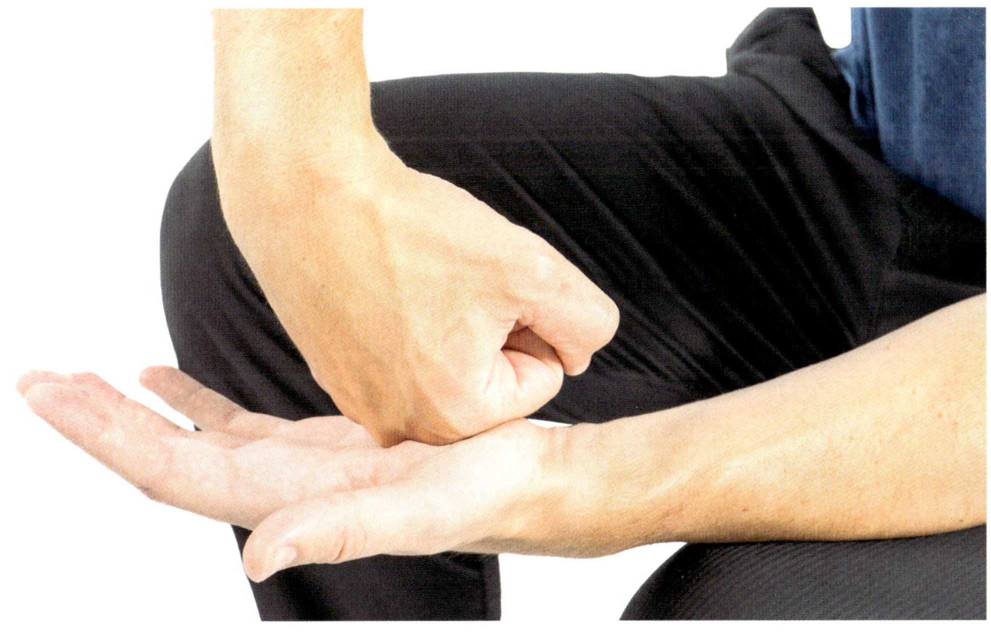

NERVE MOBILITY

MEDIAN NERVE GLIDES

Sit up tall and position your hand as if you're a waiter carrying a platter of food. Keep your wrist in that position as you slowly straighten your elbow. Once you feel like your elbow is as straight as you can get it, tilt your head in the opposite direction until you feel the slightest pull or tingle in the forearm or the middle digits. Once you feel that slight sensation, return to the starting position. Repeat this fifteen times. Ideally, you should feel both a slight relief in symptoms and an improvement in how far you were able to go. If you feel more irritated after doing these glides, you likely pushed yourself too far. Repeat this throughout the day as necessary.

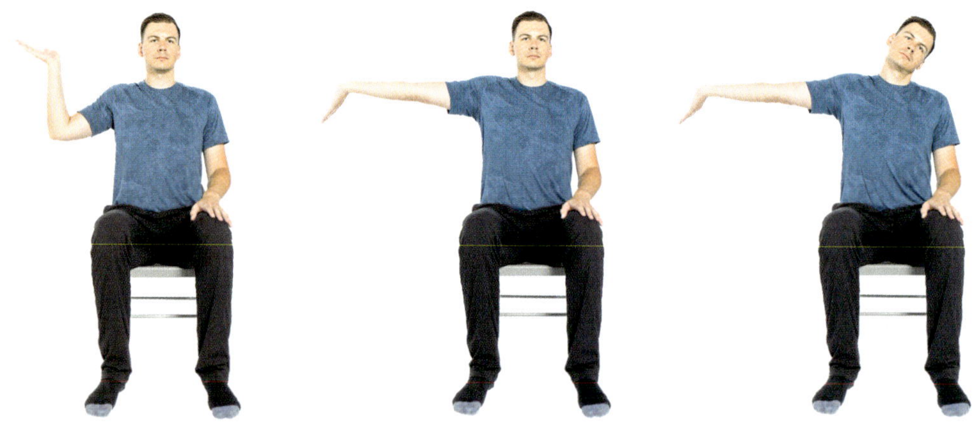

RADIAL NERVE GLIDES

Standing up tall, take the arm of the hand that you want to work on and drop it down toward the floor. Then take your hand and reach it behind you as if you were reaching for the baton in a relay race. From there, rotate your arm to the side until you feel a slight pull or tingle in the forearm or hand. Once in that position, just tilt your head in the opposite direction until you feel a slight increase in that tingle, then return to the starting position. Repeat this fifteen times. Ideally, you should feel both a slight relief in symptoms and an improvement in how far you were able to go. If you feel more irritated after doing these glides, you likely pushed yourself too far. Repeat this throughout the day as necessary.

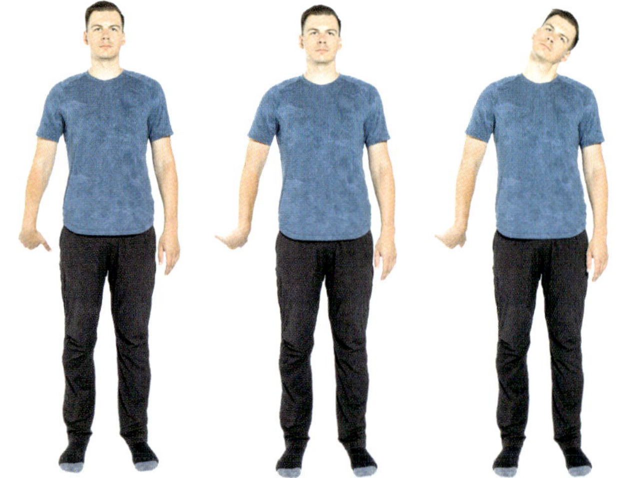

JOINT MOBILITY

WRIST JOINT GLIDES

Stand up and place your hand on a table in front of you. Then take a strap or lanyard and place it over your hand just below where the forearm ends. Slowly start to lean over your hand, taking the wrist into more extension, as you pull down on the lanyard with your opposite hand. Go until you feel a comfortable pressure, then return to the starting position. Repeat fifteen times. Soon, you will be able to comfortably go slightly further. As you repeat this over the next week or two, you should see significant improvement.

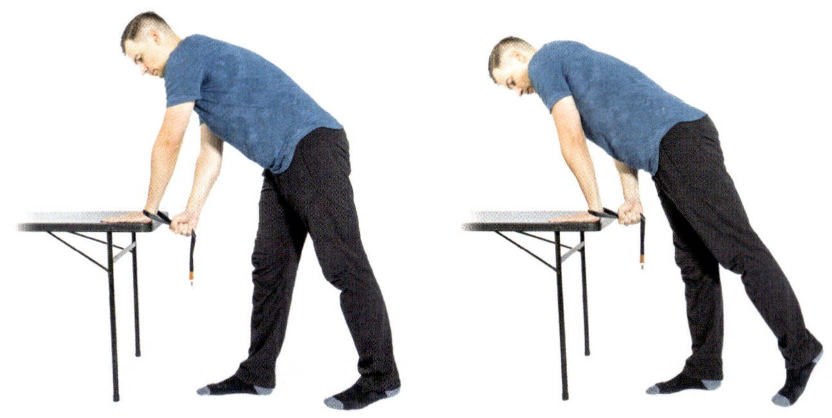

HAND STRENGTHENING

GRIP STRENGTH

There are plenty of ways to work on your grip strength, and I find it best for people to just use the technique that they are most comfortable with, whether it is squeezing some therapy putty or a stress ball or carrying a heavy weight. If you're using a ball or putty, don't go longer than three to five minutes at a time. Work on it daily, and over the course of a couple of weeks, you should see an improvement. If you opt for weights, just pick up a heavy dumbbell or kettlebell and carry it to exhaustion in sets of three. Whatever you choose, make sure that you feel fatigue in the fingers and forearm with no increase in symptoms.

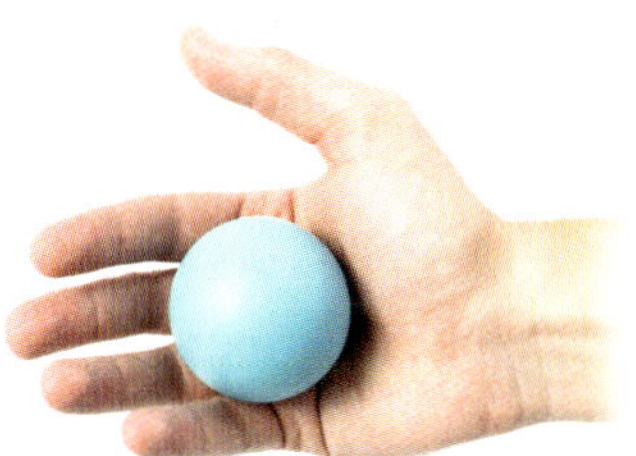

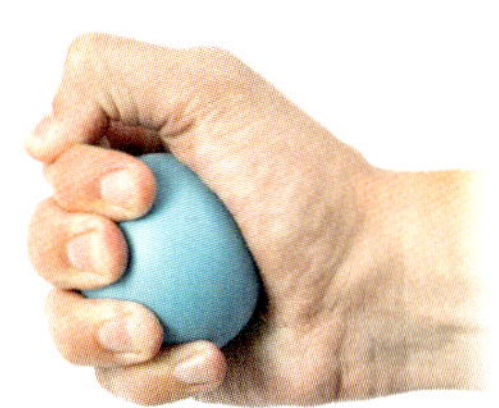

THUMB STRENGTH

Take your hand and splay it out as far as you can. Then take your thumb and reach for your first finger, trying to make the thumb travel as far as it can before having the first finger meet it. Then return to the starting position. Repeat that for the next three fingers, then work your way back to the first finger. Repeat this for two sets of ten. This is a great exercise to work on the strength of the thumb to help reduce the symptoms of De Quervain's and pollicis muscle overuse.

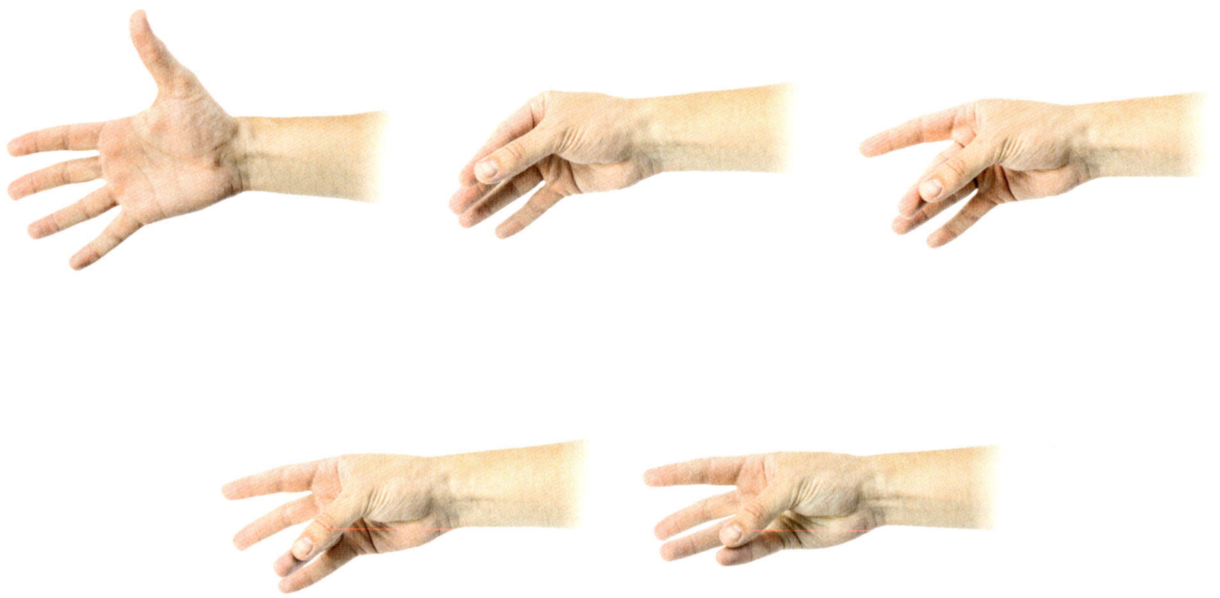

SOURCES

GENERAL ANATOMY

Gray, Henry. *Gray's Anatomy: With Original Illustrations by Henry Carter*, 42nd ed.. London, England: Arcturus Publishing, 2013.

Netter, Frank H. *Atlas of Human Anatomy*, 8th ed. Philadelphia: Elsevier, 2023.

3D4Medical. *Essential Anatomy* 5. App. Elsevier.

FOOT, ANKLE, AND LOWER LEG

American Academy of Orthopaedic Surgeons. "Stress Fractures of the Foot and Ankle." *OrthoInfo*. https://orthoinfo.aaos.org/en/diseases--conditions/stress-fractures-of-the-foot-and-ankle/.

Bhusari, N., and M. Deshmukh. "Shin Splint: A Review." *Cureus* 15, no. 1 (January 18, 2023): e33905. https://doi.org/10.7759/cureus.33905.

Chimenti, Ruth L., et al. "Achilles Pain, Stiffness, and Muscle Power Deficits: Midportion Achilles Tendinopathy Revision – 2024." *Journal of Orthopaedic & Sports Physical Therapy* 54, no. 12 (December 2024): 743–785. https://www.jospt.org/doi/10.2519/jospt.2024.0302.

Finch, P. M. "Chronic Shin Splints: A Review of the Deep Posterior Compartment." *The Foot* 8, no. 3 (1998): 119–124. https://doi.org/10.1016/S0958-2592(98)90043-8.

Martin, Robroy L., et al. "Ankle Stability and Movement Coordination Impairments: Lateral Ankle Ligament Sprains Revision 2021." *Journal of Orthopaedic & Sports Physical Therapy* 51, no. 4 (2021): CPG1–CPG32. https://www.orthopt.org/uploads/content_files/files/Ankle%20Sprain%20CPG%20Revision%202021%201.21.21%20Fig.pdf.

Melanson, S. W., and V. L. Shuman. "Acute Ankle Sprain." In *StatPearls*. Treasure Island, FL: StatPearls Publishing, 2025. https://www.ncbi.nlm.nih.gov/books/NBK459212/.

Patel, J., and M. Swords. "Hallux Rigidus." In *StatPearls*. Treasure Island, FL: StatPearls Publishing, 2025. https://www.ncbi.nlm.nih.gov/books/NBK556019/.

"Physical Therapy After an Ankle Sprain: Using the Evidence to Guide Physical Therapist Practice." *Journal of Orthopaedic & Sports Physical Therapy* 51, no. 4 (April 2021): 155–195. https://www.jospt.org/doi/10.2519/jospt.2021.0503.

Physio-Pedia. "Ottawa Ankle Rules." https://www.physiopedia.com/Ottawa_Ankle_Rules.

Smidt, K. P., and P. Massey. "5th Metatarsal Fracture." In *StatPearls*. Treasure Island, FL: StatPearls Publishing, 2025. https://www.ncbi.nlm.nih.gov/books/NBK544369/.

Washington State Department of Labor & Industries. *Foot and Ankle Guideline 2022 Updates and Corrections*. https://lni.wa.gov/patient-care/treating-patients/treatment-guidelines-and-resources/_docs/Foot_and_Ankle_Guideline_2022_updates_and_corrections.pdf.

KNEE, THIGH, AND HIP

Arundale, Amelia J.H., et al. "Exercise-Based Knee and Anterior Cruciate Ligament Injury Prevention: Clinical Practice Guidelines Linked to the International Classification of Functioning, Disability and Health." *Journal of Orthopaedic & Sports Physical Therapy* 53, no. 1 (January 2023): 1–51. https://doi.org/10.2519/jospt.2023.0301.

Bhan, K. "Meniscal Tears: Current Understanding, Diagnosis, and Management." *Cureus* 12, no. 6 (June 13, 2020): e8590. https://doi.org/10.7759/cureus.8590.

Breda, Sjouke J., et al. "Effectiveness of Progressive Tendon-Loading Exercise Therapy in Patients with Patellar Tendinopathy: A Randomised Clinical Trial." *British Journal of Sports Medicine* 55, no. 9 (2021): 501–509. https://doi.org/10.1136/bjsports-2020-102853.

Davis, D., M. Taqi, and A. Vasudevan. "Sciatica." In *StatPearls*. Treasure Island, FL: StatPearls Publishing, 2025. https://www.ncbi.nlm.nih.gov/books/NBK507908/.

Enseki, Keelan R., et al. "Hip Pain and Movement Dysfunction Associated With Nonarthritic Hip Joint Pain: A Revision." *Journal of Orthopaedic & Sports Physical Therapy* 53, no. 7 (July 2023): 375–CPG70. https://doi.org/10.2519/jospt.2023.0302.

Geng, R., et al. "Knee Osteoarthritis: Current Status and Research Progress in Treatment (Review)." *Experimental and Therapeutic Medicine* 26, no. 4 (2023): 481. https://doi.org/10.3892/etm.2023.12180.

Groh, M. M., and J. Herrera. "A Comprehensive Review of Hip Labral Tears." *Current Reviews in Musculoskeletal Medicine* 2, no. 2 (2009): 105–117. https://doi.org/10.1007/s12178-009-9052-9.

Hadeed, A., and D. C. Tapscott. "Iliotibial Band Friction Syndrome." In *StatPearls*. Treasure Island, FL: StatPearls Publishing, 2025. https://www.ncbi.nlm.nih.gov/books/NBK542185/.

Hsu, H., and R. M. Siwiec. "Knee Osteoarthritis." In *StatPearls*. Treasure Island, FL: StatPearls Publishing, 2025. https://www.ncbi.nlm.nih.gov/books/NBK507884/.

Malliaras, Peter, Jill Cook, Craig Purdam, and Ebonie Rio. "Patellar Tendinopathy: Clinical Diagnosis, Load Management, and Advice for Challenging Case Presentations." *Journal of Orthopaedic & Sports Physical Therapy* 45, no. 11 (November 2015): 887–898. https://doi.org/10.2519/jospt.2015.5987.

McKay, J., et al. "Iliotibial Band Syndrome Rehabilitation in Female Runners: A Pilot Randomized Study." *Journal of Orthopaedic Surgery and Research* 15 (2020): 188. https://doi.org/10.1186/s13018-020-01713-7.

Nasser, A. M., et al. "Proximal Hamstring Tendinopathy: A Systematic Review of Interventions." *International Journal of Sports Physical Therapy* 16, no. 2 (April 2021): 288–305. https://doi.org/10.26603/001c.21250.

Raj, M. A., and M. A. Bubnis. "Knee Meniscal Tears." In *StatPearls*. Treasure Island, FL: StatPearls Publishing, 2025. https://www.ncbi.nlm.nih.gov/books/NBK431067/.

Rio, Ebonie, et al. "Isometric Contractions Are More Analgesic Than Isotonic Contractions for Patellar Tendon Pain: An In-Season Randomized Clinical Trial." *Clinical Journal of Sport Medicine* 27, no. 3 (May 2017): 253–259. https://doi.org/10.1097/JSM.0000000000000364.

Rosen, Abigail B., et al. "Clinical Management of Patellar Tendinopathy." *Journal of Athletic Training* 57, no. 7 (July 2022): 621–631. https://doi.org/10.4085/1062-6050-0049.21.

LOWER BACK

Balza, R., and W. E. Palmer. "Symptom-Imaging Correlation in Lumbar Spine Pain." *Skeletal Radiology* 52, no. 10 (2023): 1901–1909. https://doi.org/10.1007/s00256-023-04305-8.

Brinjikji, W., et al. "Systematic Literature Review of Imaging Features of Spinal Degeneration in Asymptomatic Populations." *AJNR Am J Neuroradiol* 36, no. 4 (2015): 811–816. https://doi.org/10.3174/ajnr.A4173.

Bülow, K., et al. "General Strengthening Exercise for Chronic Low Back Pain." *Cochrane Database of Systematic Reviews* 2024, no. 3 (2024): CD015497. https://doi.org/10.1002/14651858.CD015497.

Coulombe, Bryan J., et al. "Core Stability Exercise Versus General Exercise for Chronic Low Back Pain." *Journal of Athletic Training* 52, no. 1 (2017): 71–72. https://doi.org/10.4085/1062-6050-51.11.16.

Fernández-Rodríguez, Rubén, et al. "Best Exercise Options for Reducing Pain and Disability in Adults With Chronic Low Back Pain." *Journal of Orthopaedic & Sports Physical Therapy* 52, no. 8 (2022): 505–521. https://doi.org/10.2519/jospt.2022.10671.

Flynn, Timothy W., et al. "Appropriate Use of Diagnostic Imaging in Low Back Pain." *Journal of Orthopaedic & Sports Physical Therapy* 41, no. 11 (2011): 838–846. https://doi.org/10.2519/jospt.2011.3618.

George, Steven Z., et al. "Interventions for the Management of Acute and Chronic Low Back Pain: Revision 2021." *Journal of Orthopaedic & Sports Physical Therapy* 51, no. 11 (2021): 531–550. https://doi.org/10.2519/jospt.2021.0304.

Gordon, Rebecca, and Stuart Bloxham. "A Systematic Review of the Effects of Exercise and Physical Activity on Non-Specific Chronic Low Back Pain." *Healthcare* 4, no. 2 (2016): 22. https://doi.org/10.3390/healthcare4020022.

Hayden, Jill A., et al. "Exercise Therapy for Chronic Low Back Pain." *Cochrane Database of Systematic Reviews* 9 (2021): CD009790. https://doi.org/10.1002/14651858.CD009790.pub2.

McGill, Stuart. *Back Mechanic*. 1st ed. Waterloo, ON: Stuart McGill, 2015.

McKenzie, Robin. *Treat Your Own Back*. 9th ed. Minneapolis: Orthopedic Physical Therapy Products, 2011.

MID BACK, HEAD, NECK, AND JAW

California Division of Workers' Compensation. "Cervical and Thoracic Spine Disorders." Accessed July 14, 2025. https://www.dir.ca.gov/dwc/DWCPropRegs/MTUS-Evidence-Based-Update/Guidelines/ACOEM-Cervical-and-Thoracic-Spine-Guideline.pdf.

Bednarczyk, Victoria, and Alycia Markowski. "Temporomandibular Joint Anterior Disc Displacement Without Reduction." *JOSPT Cases* 1, no. 4 (2021): 287–288. https://doi.org/10.2519/josptcases.2021.10555.

Blanpied, Peter R., et al. "Neck Pain: Revision 2017." *Journal of Orthopaedic & Sports Physical Therapy* 47, no. 7 (2017): A1–A83. https://doi.org/10.2519/jospt.2017.0302.

Harrison, Anne L., et al. "A Proposed Diagnostic Classification of Patients With Temporomandibular Disorders." *Journal of Orthopaedic & Sports Physical Therapy* 44, no. 3 (2014): 182–197. https://doi.org/10.2519/jospt.2014.4847.

Katzman, W. B., et al. "Age-Related Hyperkyphosis." *Journal of Orthopaedic & Sports Physical Therapy* 40, no. 6 (2010): 352–360. https://doi.org/10.2519/jospt.2010.3099.

Kumar, R., et al. "The Painful Rib Syndrome." *Indian Journal of Anaesthesia* 57, no. 3 (2013): 311–313. https://doi.org/10.4103/0019-5049.115585.

Lindfors, E., et al. "Jaw Exercises in the Treatment of Temporomandibular Disorders." *Journal of Oral & Facial Pain and Headache* 33, no. 4 (2019): 389–398. https://doi.org/10.11607/ofph.2359.

Peng, B., and Michael J. DePalma. "Cervical Disc Degeneration and Neck Pain." *Journal of Pain Research* 11 (2018): 2853–2857. https://doi.org/10.2147/JPR.S180018.

Petcharaporn, M., et al. "Thoracic Hyperkyphosis and the Scoliosis Research Society Outcomes Instrument." *Spine* 32, no. 20 (2007): 2226–2231. https://doi.org/10.1097/BRS.0b013e31814b1bef.

Ramirez, Michelle M., et al. "Translating the Neck Pain Clinical Guidelines Into Practice." *JOSPT Open* 3, no. 2 (2025): 99–106. https://doi.org/10.2519/josptopen.2025.0101.

Risetti, M., et al. "Management of Non-Specific Thoracic Spine Pain." *BMC Musculoskeletal Disorders* 24, no. 1 (2023): 398. https://doi.org/10.1186/s12891-023-06505-8.

Shimada, A., et al. "Effectiveness of Exercise Therapy on Pain Relief and Jaw Mobility." *Frontiers in Oral Health* 4 (2023): 1170966. https://doi.org/10.3389/froh.2023.1170966.

SHOULDER

American Heart Association. "Warning Signs of a Heart Attack." Accessed July 14, 2025. https://www.heart.org/en/health-topics/heart-attack/warning-signs-of-a-heart-attack.

Bednar, E. D., et al. "Diagnosis and Management of Little League Shoulder." *Orthopaedic Journal of Sports Medicine* 9, no. 7 (2021): 23259671211017563. https://doi.org/10.1177/23259671211017563.

Dunn, Warren R., et al. "Symptoms of Pain Do Not Correlate with Rotator Cuff Tear Severity." *Journal of Bone and Joint Surgery* 96, no. 10 (2014): 793–800. https://doi.org/10.2106/JBJS.L.01304.

Kaplan, Jordan, and Ayesha Kanwal. "Thoracic Outlet Syndrome." In *StatPearls*. Treasure Island, FL: StatPearls Publishing, 2025. https://www.ncbi.nlm.nih.gov/books/NBK557450/.

Kelley, Martin J., et al. "Clinical Practice Guidelines for Shoulder Pain." *Journal of Orthopaedic & Sports Physical Therapy* 43, no. 5 (2013): 280–351. https://doi.org/10.2519/jospt.2013.0302.

Lafrance, Simon, et al. "The Efficacy of Exercise Therapy for Rotator Cuff–Related Shoulder Pain." *Journal of Orthopaedic & Sports Physical Therapy* 54, no. 8 (2024): 499–512. https://doi.org/10.2519/jospt.2024.12453.

Lee, D. Y. L., et al. "Clinical Practice Guidelines for the Management of Atraumatic Shoulder Conditions." *BMJ Open* 11, no. 4 (2021): e048297. https://doi.org/10.1136/bmjopen-2020-048297.

May, Timothy, and Gary M. Garmel. "Rotator Cuff Injury." In *StatPearls*. Treasure Island, FL: StatPearls Publishing, 2025. https://www.ncbi.nlm.nih.gov/books/NBK547664/.

Miller, Jason E., et al. "Association of Strength Measurement with Rotator Cuff Tear." *American Journal of Physical Medicine & Rehabilitation* 95, no. 1 (2016): 47–56. https://doi.org/10.1097/PHM.0000000000000329.

ELBOW, FOREARM WRIST, AND HAND

American Academy of Orthopaedic Surgeons. "Elbow (Olecranon) Bursitis." OrthoInfo. Accessed July 14, 2025. https://orthoinfo.aaos.org/en/diseases--conditions/elbow-olecranon-bursitis/.

Anderson, Derek, et al. "A Comprehensive Review of Cubital Tunnel Syndrome." *Orthopedic Reviews* 14, no. 3 (2022): 38239. https://doi.org/10.52965/001c.38239.

Lucado, Ann M., et al. "Lateral Elbow Pain and Muscle Function Impairments." *Journal of Orthopaedic & Sports Physical Therapy* 52, no. 12 (2022): 770–836. https://doi.org/10.2519/jospt.2022.0302.

Reece, C. L., D. Li, and Adam J. Susmarski. "Medial Epicondylitis." In *StatPearls*. Treasure Island, FL: StatPearls Publishing, 2025. https://www.ncbi.nlm.nih.gov/books/NBK557869/.

Satteson, Elizabeth, and S. Craig Tannan. "De Quervain Tenosynovitis." In *StatPearls*. Treasure Island, FL: StatPearls Publishing, 2025. https://www.ncbi.nlm.nih.gov/books/NBK442005/.

Sevy, Justin O., and Richard E. Sina. "Carpal Tunnel Syndrome." In *StatPearls*. Treasure Island, FL: StatPearls Publishing, 2025. https://www.ncbi.nlm.nih.gov/books/NBK448179/.

Tom, Justin A., et al. "Diagnosis and Treatment of Triceps Tendon Injuries." *Clinical Journal of Sport Medicine* 24, no. 3 (2014): 197–204. https://doi.org/10.1097/JSM.0000000000000010.

Varacallo, Matthew A., and Scott D. Mair. "Proximal Biceps Tendinitis and Tendinopathy." In *StatPearls*. Treasure Island, FL: StatPearls Publishing, 2025. https://www.ncbi.nlm.nih.gov/books/NBK533002/.

INDEX

G

H

I

J

K

L

M

N

S

T

U

V

W–Z

ABOUT THE AUTHOR

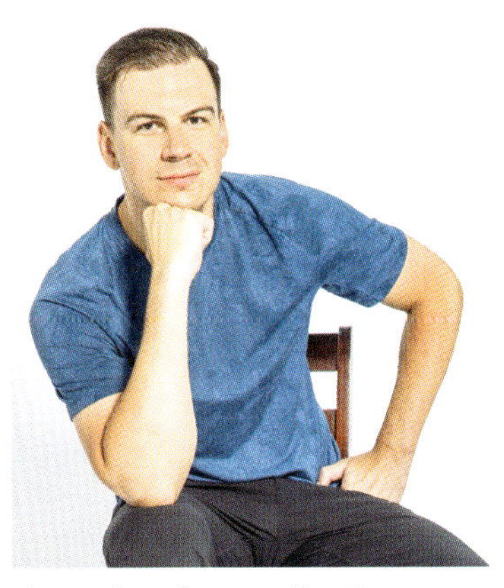

Dan Ginader is a Doctor of Physical Therapy based in Midtown Manhattan. Starting in 2020, he became widely recognized for his popular social media content explaining the common causes of aches and pains and offering simple, actionable ways to address them.

Today, with millions of followers across his platforms, Dan remains deeply committed to his in-person practice. He treats a diverse range of patients, including professional athletes and Broadway performers, as well as manual laborers and corporate professionals.

Drawing from his childhood athletic experience and a decade of care, Dan's common-sense advice looks to the roots of pain and enables his patients to understand their bodies and help themselves. His broad expertise enables him to connect with and provide effective care to people from all walks of life. Find him at @dr.dan_dpt on Instagram and on YouTube @Dr.DanDPT.